TOTAL FITNESS
THE NAUTILUS WAY

To Nick:
A good man, a true friend, and a fine person.

TOTAL FITNESS
THE NAUTILUS WAY

2nd EDITION

edited by

James A. Peterson, Ph.D.
Director of Sports Medicine
Women's Sports Foundation

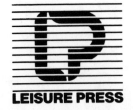

LEISURE PRESS

A publication of
Leisure Press
P.O. Box 3; West Point, N.Y. 10996

Library of Congress Catalog Card Number: 81-85623
ISBN 0-918438-40-3

PHOTO CREDITS

Bert Jacobson: 95, 159
Biz Stark: 23, 51, 71, 80, 185, 195
Bob Bertucci: 82
Chicago Cubs National League Ballclub Inc: 173, 285
Dan Riley: 102, 155
David Madison: 144
Don Gosney: 87, 132, 142, 168
Don Roberts: 49, 61, 62, 75
Ellington Darden: 108, 121, 183
Janeart, Inc.: 115, 133
John Dotson: All text photos except where credited otherwise.
Nautilus Sports/Medical Industries, Inc.: 8, 10, 13, 18, 39, 43, 45, 55, 78, 89,
    96, 100, 104, 112, 119, 125, 192, 201, 205, 213, 215, 223, 231, 281
NIRSA Journal: 84
Penn State University Sports Information Office: 151
Stanford University Sports Information Office: 139, 177, 282
Univ. of California (Men's Athletics) Sports Information Office:
    147 (David Cradeur)
University of California (Women's Athletics) Sports Information Office:
    91 (Hill), 141 (Zoller)
University of Pittsburgh Sports Information Office: 73, 136
U.S. Army Photograph: 165
Virgil Knight: 149, 155, 157, 179, 189

Text illustrations by Debra Clift.   Cover photographs by John Dotson

CONTENTS

Page

Preface 7

PART A. ARTHUR JONES — THE MAN AND HIS IDEAS

1. The History and Development of Nautilus 11
2. Exercise...Present State of the Art 21
3. What to Expect from Exercise 33
4. Progressive Exercise 47
5. Time as a Factor in Exercise 59
6. Avoiding and Preventing Injuries 67
7. Preventing Injuries in Sports 77
8. Improving Functional Ability in Any Sport 83
9. Negative Work as a Factor in Exercise 93
10. Negative Accentuated Strength Training 100
11. Metabolic Cost of Negative Work 107
12. Flexibility and Metabolic Condition 113
13. Predicting Athletic Ability 129
14. The Missing Link in Athletic Performance 137
15. The Nervous System in Sports 145
16. The Relationship of Strength to Functional Ability in Sports 163
17. Specificity in Strength Training — The Facts & Fables 169
18. Flexibility as a Result of Exercise 181
19. Increasing Neck Strength...For the Prevention of Injury 193
20. The Future of Exercise — An Opinion 199

PART B. TRAINING PRINCIPLES AND TECHNIQUES

21. Strength Training Principles (Ellington Darden) 211
22. Muscle: Structure, Function, and Control (Michael D. Wolf) 233
23. Nautilus Training (John Donati) 247
24. Strength Training: Preventive Medicine for the Athlete
    (Michael N. Fulton) 283

About the Editor 288

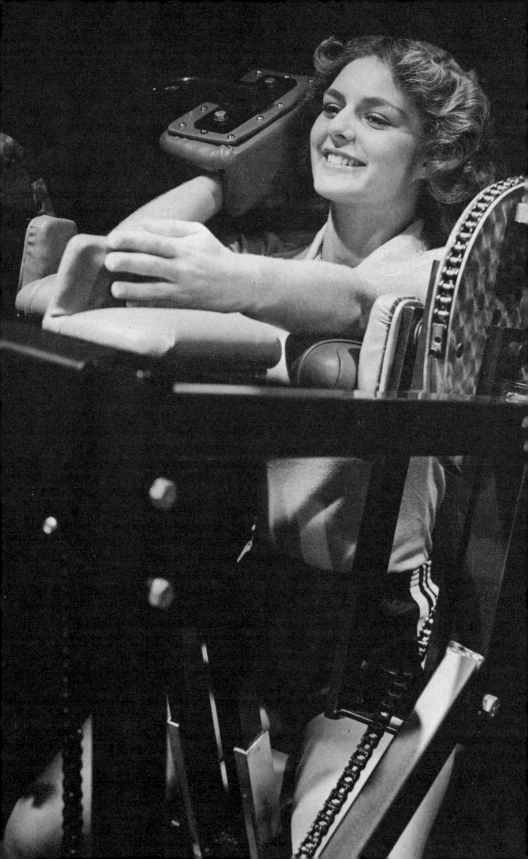

PREFACE

Everyone wants to "look fit" and "feel fit". In response to this goal, there seems to be a never-ending search for "quick fix" solutions regarding how to best develop physical fitness. New techniques, new modes of training, and new tools to train on are constantly pitched as the ultimate answer to personal conditioning. Regretably, however, most of these so-called advances are nothing more than recycled rip-offs designed to fleece a public which is frequently far too eager to obtain "an easy way to fitness". This approach is particularly evident in the area of how to develop muscular fitness. Intuition and superstition abound. "If you hurt, it must have helped you. If you worked out for a long time, you paid the proper price. If the machine you trained on is a chrome dinosaur, you obviously have the best equipment." What foolishness.

During the period 1971-1980, I had the opportunity to be directly involved with a number of research studies conducted at the United States Military Academy. Collectively, these endeavors were designed to identify the proper way to develop muscular fitness. Bit by bit, piece by piece, the information gained from these studies contributed to a 3-fold approach to training: how to develop the greatest level of strength, in the least amount of time and in the safest way possible. That approach was based upon the concept that "more is not necessarily better and that facts are more relevant than unfounded practices." Given the rigid controls that are necessary to conduct meaningful research in the area of strength training, West Point was undoubtedly the best place for undertaking such investigations.

None of this would have happened, however, without the efforts of Arthur Jones, the founder of Nautilus Sports/Medical Industries, Inc. Without his vision, willingness to provide the necessary means to conduct such research, and his unrelenting search for the truth (wherever the chips might fall), the body of knowledge relating to strength training might still rest in the dark ages. Negative-only exercise, full-range exercise, negative accentuated exercise, and infimetric exercise are but a few of the revolutionary conditioning techniques advocated, popularized, and made possible by Jones and the Nautilus equipment he designed and developed.

This second edition of **Total Fitness: The Nautilus Way** presents 25 articles on strength training. Hopefully, they will contribute to your understanding of the most effective and efficient approach to developing muscular fitness. If fitness is your goal, Nautilus is the way; not the only way, but the best way.

My appreciation is extended to John Griffith, former publisher of the **Athletic Journal** for granting permission to reprint the twenty articles by Arthur Jones from the **Athletic Journal.**

James A. Peterson, Ph.D.

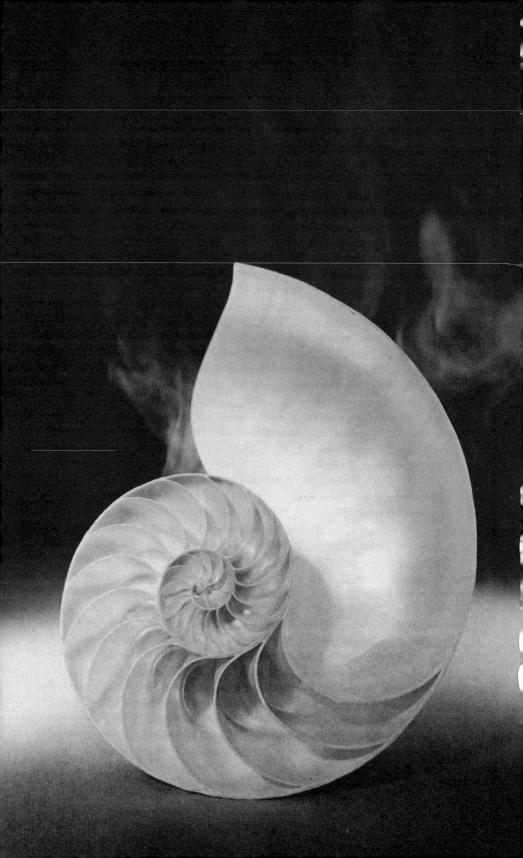

PART A

ARTHUR JONES
THE MAN AND HIS IDEAS

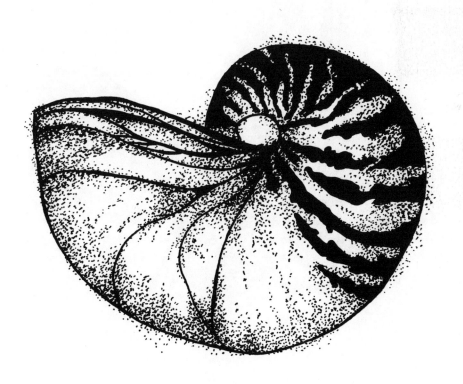

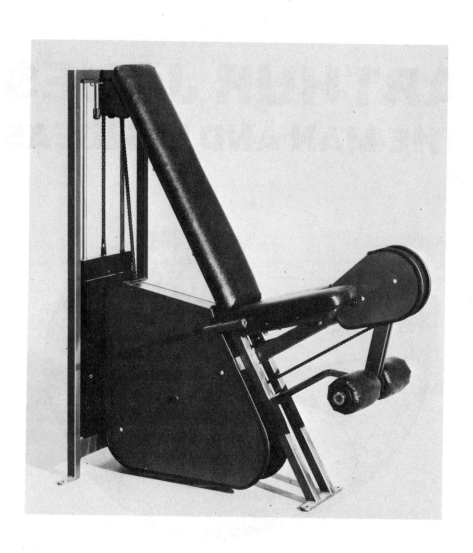

1
The History and Development of Nautilus

The first Nautilus machine was built in 1948...but the first Nautilus machine produced for sale was built more than twenty-two years later, in 1970.

The first type of machine was a Pullover Torso Machine—and the first type delivered to a customer was also a Pullover. But in fact, the two machines—the first built, and the first sold—had little more than the name in common. During the twenty-two years of developmental work that passed prior to the first sale of a Nautilus machine, twenty-seven distinct models of the Pullover were built and tested—and literally hundreds of other models were considered and rejected before reaching the prototype stage.

In short, it was a long, slow process—leading to a final result that probably would never have occurred under any other set of circumstances. The first Nautilus machine was not built for commercial purposes—instead, it was built in an attempt to produce a literally perfect exercise tool.

The first Nautilus machine was built at a time when quite a number of people were beginning to realize that something basic was missing in conventional exercises. The barbell was (and is) a tool capable of producing outstanding degrees of muscular strength—eventually; but it obviously is not the ideal tool.

At or about the same time that the first Nautilus machine was built, other people were also making attempts in the direction of improving the tools available for exercise—but they made the mistake of going in exactly the wrong direction. Instead of devoting their attentions and efforts to exercise, they concentrated on attempts to improve the available tool, the barbell.

The History and Development of Nautilus

You can design a better saddle for a horse, you can feed a horse better, you can train a horse better...but as long as you restrict your attentions to a horse, you will be forced to work within the limitations of a horse. And you will never travel faster than the maximum speed of a horse.

Modern speed of travel developed only after the horse was scrapped as a means of practical transportation.

Conventional weight machines that merely copy the functions of a barbell are now about as practical for the purpose of exercise as a horse is for the purpose of transportation.

Nautilus was based on the concept that the basic tool was wrong, so the development of Nautilus equipment was a process of determining the functions of human muscular structures—in an effort to design new and much improved tools that could meet the actual requirements of muscles. Instead of trying to fit human muscles to an imperfect tool, the barbell—Nautilus was an attempt to design perfect tools that would exactly fit the requirements of muscles.

But just what are the requirements of muscles?

To answer that question, you must first clearly understand the functions of muscles...but that is simple enough, if the problem is approached logically.

Pick a particular muscle, any particular muscle...first move into a position where the muscle you are observing is stretched into a fully extended position, where additional movement in the direction of extension is literally impossible.

Next...fully contract the same muscle, and carefully observe the resulting movement of the related body part.

Having done so, you should then be clearly aware of the movement that is produced by that particular muscle...the full range of movement, from full extension to full contraction.

If you are interested in designing an exercise to develop the strength of that particular muscle, you must build a piece of equipment that will provide constant resistance against the full range of movement—if not, then only part of that muscle will be exposed to exercise, and only part of the muscle will be developed.

One of the basic faults with the barbell is the fact that the resistance is not "direct"—instead of being directly applied to the prime body part that is actually moved by a particular muscle, the resistance is applied against a secondary body part that is "indirectly" moved.

As an unavoidable result, the muscle you are trying to work is not exposed to resistance in proportion to its own ability—instead, a point of failure is reached when a weaker muscular structure is unable to continue.

For example..."chinning" type exercises are practiced for the purpose of developing the major muscular structures of the torso, the powerful muscles of the back and chest that are attached to and move the upper arms.

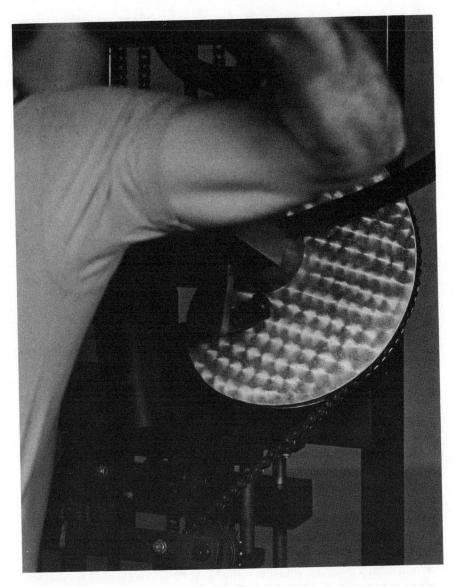

Nautilus was based on the concept that the basic tool was wrong, so the development of Nautilus equipment was a process of determining the functions of human muscular structures—in an effort to design new and much improved tools that could meet the actual requirements of muscles. Instead of trying to fit human muscles to an imperfect tool, the barbell—Nautilus was an attempt to design perfect tools that would exactly fit the requirements of muscles.

But in practice, the torso muscles are never actually exposed to heavy resistance during chinning type exercises...because the torso muscles are attached to and move the upper arms, but the resistance is not applied against the upper arms. Instead, the resistance is applied against the hands—the result being that the bending muscles of the arms are also involved in the exercise.

And since the arm muscles are smaller and weaker than the torso muscles, a point of failure is reached when the arm muscles become exhausted...and this occurs long before the larger and stronger torso muscles have been exposed to anything even approaching a proper intensity of exercise.

To exercise the muscles of the torse properly...THE RESISTANCE MUST BE APPLIED DIRECTLY AGAINST THE UPPER ARMS. In effect, against the elbows. When this is done—and ONLY when this is done—do you have "direct" resistance for the powerful muscles of the torso.

But until and unless it is done, you have only "indirect" resistance—filtered through the weak-link of the arm muscles, which will always and unavoidably limit your development during conventional exercises.

For all practical purposes, you do have "direct" resistance for the bending muscles of the arms during chinning-type exercises—and such exercises are very productive for increasing the strength of the arms. But such exercises will not—literally CANNOT—do much in the way of developing the strength of the torso muscles.

The first Nautilus machine was built in an attempt to solve that exact problem...in an effort to provide "direct" resistance for the torso muscles, while removing the involvement of the arm muscles.

Obviously, the resistance had to be applied directly against the upper arms, the elbows...and this was done. But doing so involved the design and construction of a machine that would provide a rotary form of resistance—since the resulting movement of the elbows is rotary in nature.

So the first basic requirement for a perfect exercise for the muscles of the torso was "direct" resistance—applied against the elbows.

And the second basic requirement was a rotary form of resistance—rotating on a common axis with the upper arms, rotating around the axis of the shoulder joints.

When such a machine was first built, it was immediately obvious that we had gone a great distance in the right direction...but it was equally obvious that a lot more remained to be done.

For one thing, we then became clearly aware that "constant" resistance was not enough...because you are much stronger in some positions than you are in other positions. So the resistance had to change during the actual movement.

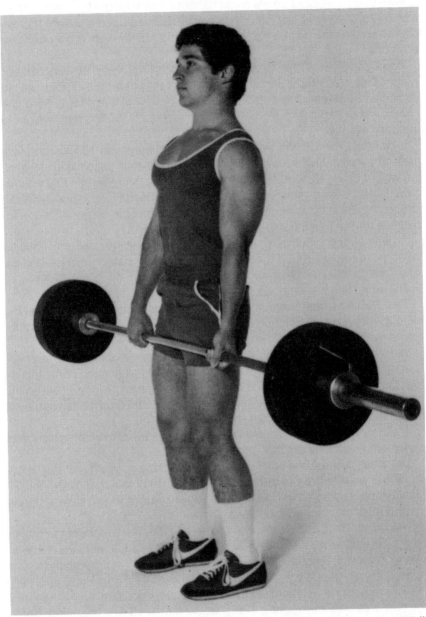

One of the basic faults with the barbell is the fact that the resistance is not "direct"—instead of being directly applied to the prime body part that is actually moved by a particular muscle, the resistance is applied against a secondary body part that is "indirectly" moved.

If we used a weight that we could handle in our strongest position, then it was far too heavy in any other position...and if we used a weight that we could handle in our weakest position, then it was far too light in our strongest positions.

Twenty-five years ago, we first approached this problem by using a basic weight that was proper for use in our weakest position...but then we attached a number of chains to the base weight. As the weight was lifted, the chains were gradually pulled off the floor—steadily adding their weight to the base weight.

It worked...even if not perfectly. But it certainly was NOT a practical method of regulating the weight. And while it was thus possible to increase the weight at any desired rate...we could not then decrease it if that was required. And it was required; because, in most situations, your available strength increases with movement in the direction of contraction...increases up to a point, but then decreases.

So we needed a method of regulating the resistance that would permit us to increase the weight up to a certain point and then decrease it—and we could not do that with chains.

Thus the Nautilus "cam" was born.

The Nautilus cam regulates the resistance automatically, instantly, exactly...providing resistance that meets the basic requirements of proper exercise in all positions.

In a typical situation...at the start of the movement your available strength is at its lowest level, so the radius of the cam is small and the resistance is low. But as you move into another position your strength increases, so the radius of the cam becomes larger in proportion—and thus the resistance is increased to match your higher strength level.

When you reach your strongest position, the radius of the cam is also at its maximum—and thus the resistance is maximum.

Then, as you pass the point of greatest available strength and start moving into a weaker area of movement...the radius of the cam automatically and instantly reduces itself in exact proportion, thus reducing the resistance in proportion to your declining strength.

The actual resistance is thus changing constantly throughout the movement...but it doesn't "feel" like it is changing. Instead, it feels the same in every position. It feels the same because it is always in proportion to your available strength.

If the resistance was actually the same in every position, as it would be if the cam was perfectly round...then it would feel like it was changing. But in such a case it wouldn't be the resistance that was changing...instead it would be your strength that was changing.

To make this point perfectly clear to visitors with little knowledge of basic physics...we had, until recently, a very early model Nautilus Pullover Machine that actually had round pulleys instead of eccentric cams. Thus this machine had constant and even resistance.

Seated in this machine, and belted in, a visitor would be given a weight that he could easily handle in his strongest position...and it would feel very light to him, in that position.

But then we would tell him to let the weight pull him back in the direction of an extended position...and as he moved, the same weight would start to feel much heavier. After about sixty degrees of rotary movement, the weight would feel VERY HEAVY...and the visitor would suddenly realize that the weight was far too heavy for him to stop the movement. It would appear that a weight which had been light in his strongest position was now going to tear his upper arms out by their roots.

And it would...except, at that point, we removed the weight. Such a demonstration is of far more value than a million words of explanation. Because an explanation may or may not be understood—but such an example can be experienced, can be felt, cannot be denied.

Such a demonstration makes you clearly aware of the absolute REQUIREMENT for valuable resistance, for resistance that changes instantly and automatically as you move during an exercise.

You may understand that such a requirement exists...but it is very unlikely that you will fully appreciate the enormous IMPORTANCE of such variable resistance until you experience a full range, direct exercise that does not have variable resistance.

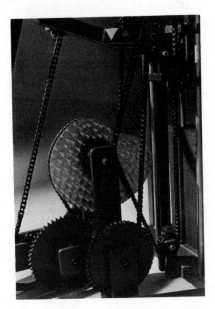

The Nautilus cam regulates the resistance automatically, instantly, exactly...providing resistance that meets your requirements in all positions.

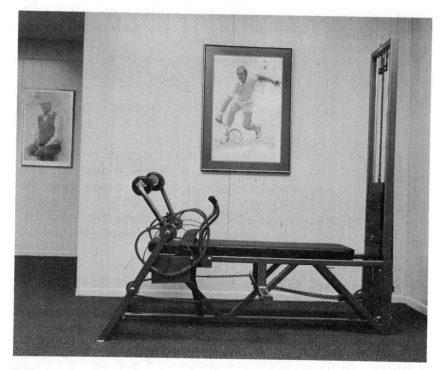

There is absolutely nothing 'random' about the design of a Nautilus machine..."function dictates design," and the functions demanded by a perfect form of exercise dictate the design of Nautilus machines.

You probably understand the advantage of round wheels on your car—but it is unlikely that you will fully appreciate round wheels until and unless you try driving a car with square wheels. After which experience, any lingering doubts about the requirement for round wheels will be permanently removed from your mind.

Many of the features incorporated into the design of Nautilus machines are not fully appreciated by people...until they experience a full range, direct exercise that does not provide those features.

For example...the mass of the "resistance arms" is counter-weighted in such a manner that it is perfectly balanced, effectively weighing literally nothing. In the Pullover Machine, this mass would add a total of 383.25 "inch pounds" of torque to the resistance in some areas of the movement—and would subtract an equal amount of resistance in other areas of movement—and would disrupt the variation of resistance throughout the movement.

In some places, this uncontrolled mass would "help" you—in other areas of movement it would "hurt" you—and in all areas of movement it would make exact regulation of the resistance impossible.

So it MUST BE BALANCED OUT—and when it has been balanced out, then you might not fully appreciate just how important a requirement that really is unless you tried a machine that had NOT been counter-weighed.

In the combination Pullover and Torso/Arm Machine, the required counter-weight "club" weighs 52-1/2 pounds—and one of the sprockets that drives this counter-weight weighs 23 pounds—and the heavy double chain has a test strength of 7,400 pounds. All of which size and strength of construction is REQUIRED.

In that machine, the counter-weight is "timed" like an automobile ignition system...it must be, in order that it will always exactly "balance out" the mass of the resistance-arm during a full 240 degrees of rotary movement.

Without this counter-weight system...the resistance would be much too heavy in the starting position—and too light in the finishing position, and FAR TOO LIGHT in the position where you are strongest.

If you remove the counter-weight from a machine, the exercise performed on that machine will then feel like an entirely different exercise—because it would be an entirely different, unbalanced exercise.

There is absolutely nothing "random" about the design of a Nautilus machine..."function dictates design," and the functions demanded by a perfect form of exercise dictate the design of Nautilus machines.

Over a period of more than twenty years we gradually became clearly aware of all of the requirements for a perfect form of exercise...these requirements are...

- Full-range resistance
- Direct resistance
- Balanced resistance
- Omni-directional resistance
- Automatically-variable resistance
- Rotary-form resistance
- Negative-work potential

Conventional exercises provide only one of those absolute requirements (negative-work potential) and thus conventional exercises are NOT full-range exercises, are NOT proper exercises, are nowhere near as productive as they should be in proportion to the amount of time and effort devoted to them.

Isokinetic exercises have NONE of these features—and thus Isokinetic resistance is the least productive form of exercise for any purpose.

Nautilus provides all of these requirements. Nautilus is the ONLY full-range exercise. Nautilus is the ONLY source of "total" exercise.

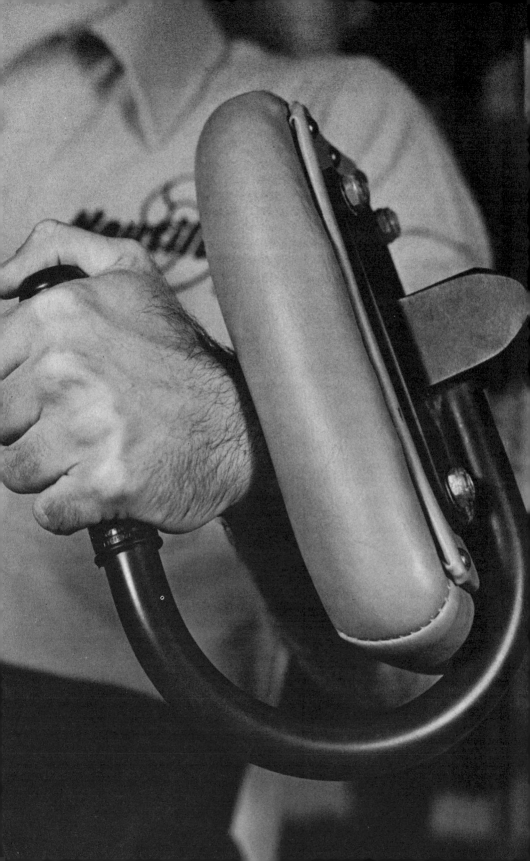

2
EXERCISE...
Present State of the Art

By Arthur Jones

The *Pullover Torso Machine was the first Nautilus* machine, the second, and the third...its development extended over a period of twenty-two years, and the first machine delivered to a customer was the twenty-seventh model. The exclusive features now incorporated in all *Nautilus* machines were outgrowths of the long, slow development of the *Pullover* machine.

Certain basic features were required for the development of a practical airplane...lift, thrust, and three-axis control...and until these requirements were understood and provided, the airplane remained a dream. Today, all airplanes incorporate these same three basic features...as they must. The airplane is not the only means of transportation, but it certainly is the fastest.

Early attempts to build an airplane failed because the builders did not understand the basic requirements of flight...today, many forms of exercise fail for much the same reason, because the designers of the equipment do not understand the basic requirements for productive exercise.

If an airplane fails to fly, its failure is immediately obvious...and the market for such an attempt at flight is zero, so our airports are not cluttered with thousands of unsuccessful airplanes, failures.

If the requirements for productive exercise are clearly understood, then it is just as easy to recognize an unsuccessful form of exercise...yet literally millions of worthless and near-worthless exercise devices are cluttering the homes and gymnasiums in this country alone. Many people do not understand the basic requirements.

Used properly, a barbell is capable of safely producing worthwhile results...the problem arises from the fact that very few people use a barbell properly. But even when it is used properly, a barbell has certain definite limitations. So if the value of a barbell is clearly understood, and if the limitations are also understood, then it becomes possible to take the next step...an evolutionary step, a step up to a type of equipment that provides the actual value of a barbell without the limitations.

Just what is the actual *value* of a barbell? It provides heavy resistance against the movement produced by muscular contraction. What are the limitations of a barbell? Resistance is *not* provided against full-range movement.

Serious attempts in the direction of solving the problems involved in providing full-range exercise for the muscles of the torso were first undertaken in 1948...and the first truly practical *Pullover Torso Machine* was built in 1967, nineteen years later.

In the meantime, other people were working on similar problems...from another angle, which led to the development of the *Universal* type exercise machines. Resistance was provided in the form of self-contained, quick-change, pin-selector type weight stacks. It was no longer necessary to add or remove barbell plates. Instead, the required amount of resistance could be provided by moving a pin from one hole to another...so the speed of use, and thus the convenience, was greatly increased.

Resistance was *redirected* from the vertical *up and down* direction provided by a barbell...this use of pulleys made it possible to perform exercises that were difficult or impossible to perform with a barbell. The resistance was *guided* by the use of guide-rods...removing the requirement for balance that is involved in almost all barbell exercises.

These features, in general, were improvements...but they were primarily improvements in convenience and safety. Little or nothing was done in the way of improving the results of such exercise...and an equal degree of results could still be produced by a barbell. In some cases, a barbell would produce better results.

Such exercises, however, still had all of the same problems encountered in barbell exercises—particularly those relating to how the resistance was being provided. The resistance was still *indirectly* applied to secondary body parts, instead of being directly applied to the prime body part...the resistance was still *straight line* in nature, instead of rotating on a common axis with the involved joints...the resistance still varied in a random manner as a result of changing leverage, instead of variation in proportion to available strength...sticking points were still encountered...areas of little or no resistance were still involved. In short...*full-range exercise was not provided.*

A few attempts at providing a rotary form of resistance were made...the leg extension machine being one example, and the leg-curl machine being another. But even a casual examination of these machines makes it im-

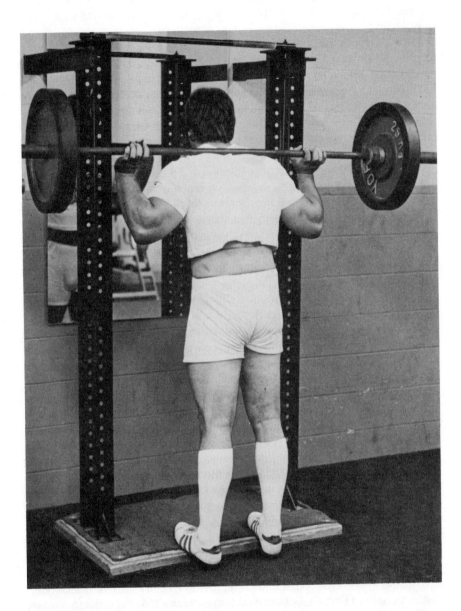

Just what is the actual value of a barbell? It provides heavy resistance against the movement produced by muscular contraction. What is the primary limitation of a barbell? Resistance is not provided against full-range movement.

mediately obvious that the designers simply did not understand the requirements. The leg extension machine is a perfect example of this lack of understanding.

In general appearance, at first glance...the leg extension machine seems to provide a rotary form of exercise, but look closer, appearances can be misleading...and in this case, they are.

The resistance is *directly* applied to the prime body part, the lower legs, as it should be...so far, so good, this is a start in the right direction. The axis of rotation of the machine is situated in line with the axis of the knees, as it should be...another step in the right direction. At that point the design went astray.

Two sources of resistance are provided in a leg extension machine. The primary source of resistance is a built-in stack of weights...and this resistance is directed against the movement-arm of the machine by a series of pulleys. The pulleys are directed in such a way that the *direction of pull* is approximately horizontal, parallel with the floor. The result is that *direct* resistance is provided only at the start of the movement.

And...as the direction of movement changes, as it must, the resulting change in the direction of the pull of the resistance causes the amount of resistance to drop off rapidly. In effect, the resistance is heavy at the start of the movement...and then becomes lighter at the end of the movement.

However...a secondary source of resistance is provided in the form of a horn on the front of the movement-arm, a pin placed there for the purpose of holding additional resistance in the form of barbell plates. The geometry of this resistance source is exactly backward to the primary resistance source. Barbell plates added to the pin provide position...and provide direct resistance only in the finishing position.

So the evolutionary development of this machine is obvious. It was built first with only one resistance source, the weight stack...but when it was seen that the weight stack did not provide enough resistance for this exercise, it was decided to add more resistance in the form of barbell plates.

It is just as obvious that the designers of the machine remained unaware of the fact that one source of resistance was providing *increasing* resistance while the other source was providing *decreasing* resistance.

Rotary movement is not enough...there must also be a rotary form of resistance against that movement. The leg extension machine provides rotary movement for the lower legs, and it directly applies the resistance against the lower legs...but it does not provide a rotary form of resistance.

A man named Bob Clark built a curling machine that did provide a rotary form of resistance, so it went a step further in the right direction...but again it failed, because it was based on a round pulley. The resistance was direct and constant throughout the movement...all well and good, but it did not vary in proportion to the exerciser's changing strength in various positions. The resistance was thus far too heavy at the start of the movement and too light at every other point in the movement.

The so-called *butterfly* machine was another attempt in the direction of providing rotary form, full-range exercise...but it failed also, for the same reason that Clark's curling machine failed, and for another reason. It also failed because the location of the arm pads literally prevented a full-range movement. The pads prevented the user from reaching a position of full muscular contraction.

So we were certainly not the only people who were aware of the shortcomings of barbell exercises, and a long list of exercise machines and devices have been built by a number of people...but if the results of the developmental work on the part of other people are any clue to their knowledge, then it is obvious that their thinking is still being limited by the same problems encountered in barbell exercises.

A clear understanding of the requirements for truly full-range exercise did not come to us in a moment of flashing insight either...instead, it was a long, slow process.

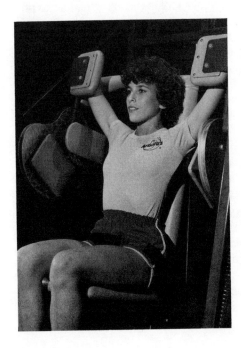

Rotary movement is not enough ...there must also be a rotary form of resistance against the movement.

Exercise...Present State of the Art

The *Pullover Torso Machine* was the first result of our growing knowledge of the actual requirements for full-range exericse...and, once those requirements were understood, and the related problems were understood, and the related problems were solved, it then became possible to apply the same principles to the development of almost any muscular structure.

The mechanical problems were somewhat different in each individual case, but the basic principles remained the same...all muscles function in the same manner, producing movement of a related body part by contraction, so the requirements for muscular development are the same regardless of which muscle is involved.

Then along came isokinetics. The claims made on behalf of isokinetic exercise were many and varied...1) it provides full-range exercise...2) it provides a higher intensity of muscular contraction...3) it provides a very safe form of exercise. None of the above three claims is true, for obvious reasons.

Full-range exercise is utterly impossible without the back pressure of a force pulling against the user's muscles prior to the start of movement. Full-range exercise is also impossible without resistance in the fully contracted position at the end of an exercise movement. Isokinetic exercises do not have back pressure...and thus stretching of the joints and pre-stretching of the involved muscles is not provided by such a form of exercise. Second, without back pressure there is no resistance in the position of full muscular contraction at the end of an exercise...again, isokinetic exercise fails to provide this requirement. In fact...since there is not resistance at either end of a movement, isokinetic exercise obviously is not a full-range form of exercise.

The next claim...that isokinetic exercise provides a higher level of intensity. This is also invalid, and for the same reason, because there is no back pressure at the start of a movement...back pressure that is required for pre-stretching the involved muscles. It is a well-established fact that pre-stretching of a muscle is required for a maximum muscular contraction. So again the claim is false.

The final claim...that isokinetic resistance provides the safest form of exercise. In fact, it is probably the most dangerous form of exercise for two reasons...1) because it results in greatly elevated blood pressure...and 2) because the involved forces are far higher than either necessary or desirable. Or, at least, the forces will be higher if the user performs the exercises in the manner suggested by the makers of isokinetic devices.

Therefore, all of the first three claims are patently false, and obviously untrue...but some of the other claims being made in regard to isokinetic exercises are true.

For example, it is claimed that such exercises produce little or nothing in the way of muscular soreness...and this lack of resulting soreness is attributed to the fact that isokinetic exercises involve no eccentric contraction (negative work). Both of those statements are true...but they certainly are not advantages. The total lack of negative work is the very root of most of the problems encountered in isokinetic exercises.

Negative work provides stretching...negative work provides pre-stretching...negative work provides resistance in the position of full muscular contraction. Without the back pressure that produces negative work, full-range exercise is *impossible*.

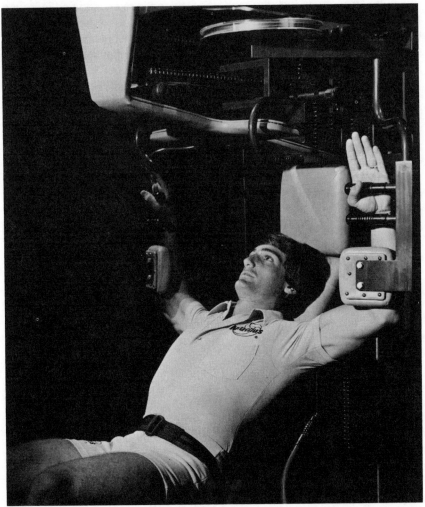

Full-range exercise is utterly impossible without the back pressure of a force pulling against the user's muscles prior to the start of movement.

Obviously, being aware of this major shortcoming in their exercises, the makers of isokinetic devices engaged in a massive advertising program in an attempt to convince the public that negative work was somehow bad...of no value, to be avoided, and dangerous.

After reading such statements for a year or so, and being aware of the actual facts all the time...we decided to run some tests to determine which forms of training actually provide both negative and positive work.

When these tests were conducted, it was obvious that negative work is actually the most important part of exercise...for the purpose of increasing muscular strength. In fact, the makers of isokinetic exercises had removed the most important part of exercise...and then pointed to the results as an improvement. This is not meant to imply that positive work has no value as a part of exercise...it certainly does, but it is not as important as negative work for the purpose of increasing strength.

Remember...full-range exercise is impossible without negative work. Not difficult...not less productive...utterly *impossible*. Negative work does result in muscular soreness when used by a previously untrained individual...but this is apparently the unavoidable price of worthwhile results. In any case, the soreness will be gone in two or three days...and it will not return as long as the athlete continues his training on a fairly regular basis.

An isokinetic form of resistance could easily be incorporated into the machines we designed...and doing so would reduce the weight, the complexity, and the cost of the machines, thus providing a much larger market. But this will never be done...because using an isokinetic form of resistance requires the total removal of negative work. The result is a mid-range, positive-only form of exercise with very little value.

The only real advantage provided by isokinetic resistance is the fact that it does not require a heavy and expensive stack of weights...instead of weights, a simple and relatively inexpensive friction device is used. This *advantage*, of course, is purchased at the price of almost total destruction of the function...so it is clearly no bargain, not even a compromise worthy of consideration.

Then...along came INFItonic and INFImetric exercise. This is a totally new form of exercise that does not involve the use of weights...a form of exercise that uses no resistance source of any kind...yet a form of exercise that requires no compromise...a form of exercise that provides all of the requirements for truly full-range exercise...while actually improving the production of results.

Any really productive form of exercise provides both positive and negative work...with a barbell the user performs positive work while lifting the weight and negative work while lowering the weight.

During the performance of standing presses with a barbell, the user performs positive work with both arms whlie raising the weight...then performs negative work with both arms while lowering the weight back to his chest. *And*...if the speed of movement is steady while both raising and lowering the weight, the forces are exactly the same in both cases.

With a pair of dumbbells, it is possible to press one dumbbell overhead while lowering the other dumbbell back to the shoulder...thus one arm is performing positive work while the other arm is performing negative work. In a manner of speaking, we might say that one arm is *doing work* while the other arm is *undoing work*.

If the movement of the two dumbbells is perfectly synchronized...if one dumbbell reaches the top position at exactly the same time that the other dumbbell reaches the bottom position...and if both dumbbells reach the mid-point of movement at the same time...then, in effect and in fact, the net balance of work that has been performed at any given moment is literally *zero*.

This being true, and it is true...then why are weights needed at all? *In fact*...weights are not needed. An exerciser does not need any source of resistance.

Or, at least...when the implications are clearly understood, then it becomes possible to design a perfect form of exercise without any external source of resistance. This perfect form of exercise consists of full-range movement against constant resistance...with both negative and positive work...with both stretching for increased flexibility and pre-stretching for high-intensity of muscular contraction...with resistance in the position of full muscular contraction.

The only change that is involved is a change from *two-limb movement* to alternate *one-limb movement*...in effect, an athlete cannot perform either positive or negative work with both arms (or legs) at the same time...instead, he must perform positive work with one arm (or leg) while he is performing negative work with the other arm (or leg). *Because*...the arm (or leg) that is performing negative work is providing the resistance for the arm (or leg) that is performing positive work, and vice versa.

Human muscles are capable of working with more resistance while performing negative work...in effect, an exerciser can lower more weight than he can lift. But in almost all forms of exercise that fact has not the slightest effect upon the exercise itself...because an exerciser is always limited by the strength that is available for positive work. He *could* lower more weight under full control...if he could lift it...but he cannot lift it, so the momentary level of his positive strength serves as a limiting factor for both his positive and negative work.

Thus...if both the positive and negative parts of the exercise are performed properly, in good form...then the forces involved in the positive part will be exactly equal to the forces involved in the negative part. This is true with a barbell, with a *Universal* type machine, and with most of the machines we designed.

This being true, as it is...it should then be obvious that the forces (both positive and negative) in INFItonic—INFImetric exercise are in no way different from the forces involved in most other exercises.

And in practice...they may well be better. Many people pay careful attention to the *lifting* part of their exercises (the positive work)...then drop the weight back down in a very sloppy fashion, thus depriving themselves of the most productive part of the exercise, the negative work.

However...with INFItonic—INFImetric exercises, the form must be good during both the positive and negative parts of the movement, because the positive work provides the negative resistance...and the negative work provides the positive resistance. Literally, an exerciser cannot have one without the other.

Isokinetic exercises, in addition to all of their other problems and shortcomings, are limited to a particular, pre-set speed of movement...a limitation which is *not* encountered in INFItonic—INFImetric exercises. An exerciser can move as fast as possible, as slow as he chooses...or at any speed between *zero speed* and maximum speed.

Another advantage to be found in this form of exercise results from the fact that the movements must be performed alternately. This style of performance makes *cheating* almost impossible...since the exerciser's limbs are moving in opposite directions, good posture (and good form) is a requirement.

And...such a style of performance also makes it possible to move into positions that would normally be impossible. For example, in a normal bench-press, contraction of the pectoral muscles is limited by the fact that the exerciser's hands must remain fairly wide-spread in the finishing position...but in an INFItonic—INFImetric bench press, the arms can actually cross above the chest, thus allowing full contraction of the pectoral muscles during a bench-press. This is possible because both arms are not in the contracted position at the same time.

All of the normal features of *Nautilus* machines are still required...the resistance must still be directly applied against the prime body part...the resistance must still rotate on a common axis with the involved joint...and the resistance must still be varied automatically and instantly in accord with the exerciser's available strength in all positions throughout a full-range of possible movement.

All that has really been done (quite a lot, as it happens) is to remove the requirement for a weight stack...and make the machines easier to enter.

What effect will this new form of exercise have on the production and sale of the regular line of the newest type of exercise machines? Probably little or no effect for a period of at least several years...because the regular line of these machines is just as good if properly used, and because it will take most people quite a long time to accept the fact that weights are actually no longer required.

Remember...in the minds of many people, the *means has become an end*. They like to see the weights go up and down...without weights, it will be hard to convince them that exercise is being provided. Eventually, some time in the probably distant future, weights will become a thing of the past...in any form.

If an athlete is building strength *in order to lift weights*...then he will have to continue lifting weights in order to develop the required style if for no other reason. But if he is lifting weights to build strength, then weights are no longer required...better results can be produced without them.

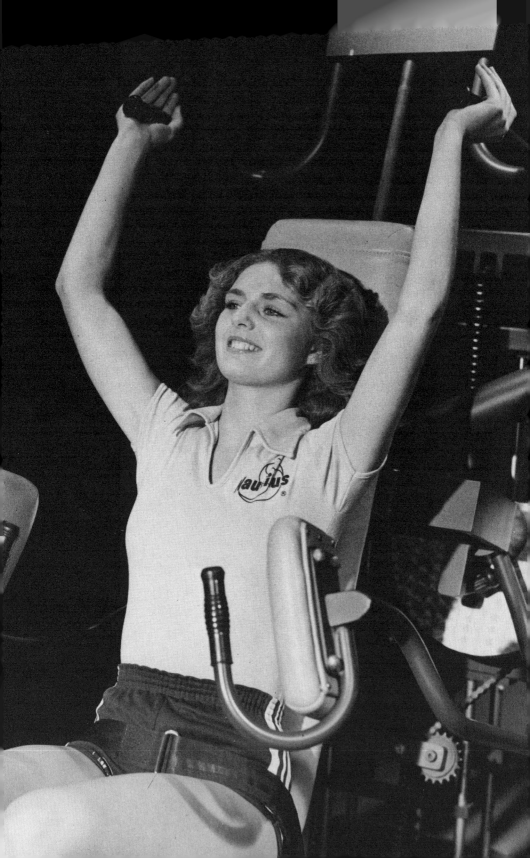

3
What to Expect from Exercise

By Arthur Jones

Eugene "Mercury" Morris of the Miami Dolphins professional football team is a product of heavy, progressive exercise. At a body weight far below the average in professional football, he is one of the strongest athletes in the history of that sport and one of the fastest. His strength and his speed are in large part direct results of exercise—proper exercise.

When Morris reported to the Dolphins' training camp in 1973, he was approximately 7 pounds heavier than he was a year earlier, but at a body weight of 197, he was stronger than he ever was before, and faster. During pre-season trials, he ran the fastest 40-yard dash in his career. Some people might feel that he was faster in spite of his increased body weight. In fact, he was faster *because of his increased body weight.*

This is not always the case. If Morris were a gymnast, for example, then increased body weight might, or might not, be an advantage, depending primarily upon where the body weight was added. Stronger, and thus larger and heavier, torso and arm muscles might help the performance of a gymnast, but with the exception of floor exercise, heavier legs would almost certainly hurt his performance.

Increasing the strength of a conditioned athlete almost always involves an increase in body weight. In some cases, this is an advantage; in other cases it is an unnecessary burden that adds nothing to the performance ability.

There is certainly no implication that exercise should not be used as a part of a gymnast's training; on the contrary, it should be. Heavy, progressive exercise should form an important part of the training of *all* athletes in *every* sport.

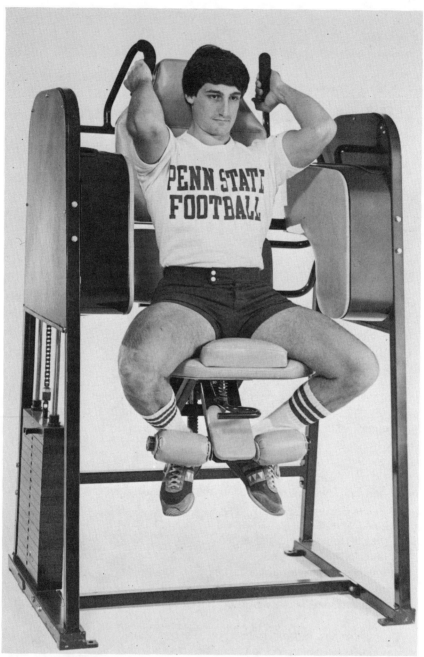

Heavy, progressive exercise should form an important part of the training of all athletes in every sport.

What to Expect from Exercise

Properly performed exercise will improve the condition, the overall system of any athlete. The conditioning results of exercise are produced regardless of what part of the muscular structure is being exercised. Working the arms has exactly the same effect on the heart and lungs as exercise involving the legs if the total amount of work and the pace are the same. The heart and lungs do not know which muscles are working. Foot-pounds of work performed and the pace of training are all that matter for conditioning purposes.

But strength increases are specific to a high degree. Heavy exercise performed for the right arm will do very little for the left arm and almost nothing for the legs. While it is true that some degree of *lateral effect* does occur, it is very limited in its results. *Lateral effect* is growth produced in, for example, an unworked left arm by exercise peformed by the right arm.

It is also true that an even greater degree of *indirect effect* is also produced by exercise. But again, it is limited in its results. *Indirect effect* is growth produced in one muscular structure as a result of exercise performed by other muscles.

However, if we accept the limited results of lateral effect and indirect effect, then the strength increases resulting from exercxise are almost entirely specific in nature. Work must be performed by the muscle the athlete is attempting to strengthen.

For our purposes it is safe to assume that the conditioning results of exercise are *general* and the strength increasing results are *specific*.

All athletes need conditioning exercises, although some sports require much higher levels of conditioning and all athetes need strength-building exercises. But in all sports activities, the training must be tailored to the requirements of the individual.

It must be clearly understood that we are dealing not only with the requirements of a particular sport, but also with the requirements of an individual athlete. The goals should be, and the possible results from exercise are: 1) a level of condition required by the particular sport; 2) maximum strength in all of the muscular structures involved in that sport; 3) at least a reasonable level of strength in all of the muscular structures of the body; and 4) maximum possible flexibility.

When those four goals have been reached, then the coach has accomplished all the exercise is capable of doing for a healthy athlete, a great deal more than most coaches suspect.

Do not expect exercise to turn an inferior athlete into a super athlete. Proper exercise will improve any athlete, and will imrove some athletes to a degree that must literally be seen to be believed; but it cannot change bodily leverage, cannot improve reaction time and it cannot give an individual the judgment required by an outstanding athlete.

What to Expect from Exercise

At some point in the distant future, coaches will look back on present athletic training practices as the *dark ages* of sport, and will seriously wonder how any athlete survived several years of professional sport without permanent injury. Quite honestly, there are not many players who do not sustain a permanent injury. Within the last year we have heard two supposedly informal estimates of the number of serious knee injuries resulting from each year of football at all levels. One estimate was 23,000 and the other was 63,000. Regardless of the actual number, it is far too high, and to a large degree unnecessary. Many such injuries could be prevented by proper exercise.

Future large-scale improvements in training practices will come primarily from a better understanding of exercise but such improvements will not come soon.

At the present time most coaches are finally becoming aware that exercise offers something of value, but very few coaches have any real idea of the actual value of exercise, and even fewer know how to go about producing those results they are seeking.

A coach can make his athletes stronger, faster, and he can greatly reduce the chances of injury. This series of articles will tell exactly how to go about producing those results, step by step, in simple terms.

Repetition is unavoidable, and in any case, it is a required part of the learning process so there will be a great deal of repetition throughout this series of articles. In particular, coaches will be told repeatedly to have their athletes *train harder,* and *train less.* But repetition is necessary to make coaches understand exactly what is meant by *hard training* and repeated examples are required to make them accept the fact that a *large amount* of training is neither necessary nor desirable.

The entire field of exercise still suffers, and it suffers badly from the old myths that have survived from the last century. Such myths must be exposed and they will be, but this also requires repetition. As long as any of the old myths still linger in a coach's mind, he will deny himself and the athletes under his control at least part of the potentially great advantages of exercise.

Coaches can expect a great deal from exercise, probably far more than they suspect. They should expect a great deal and if their training is conducted properly, the results will almost certainly exceed their highest expectations.

The Correct Amount of Exercise

How much exercise is enough? The minimum that will produce the desired result should be used. Any exercise in excess of the minimum amount *required* will be wasted effort at best and counter-productive at the worst. For an athlete too much exercise may well be worse than no exercise at all.

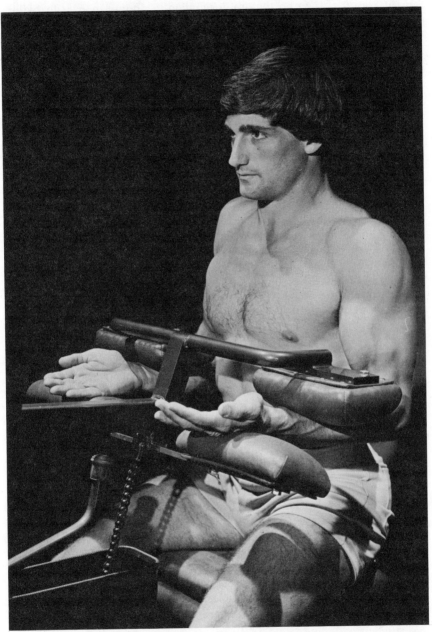

How much exercise is enough? The minimum that will produce the desired result should be used. Any exercise in excess of the minimum amount required
will be wasted effort at best and counter-productive at the worst.

Simply from the apparent natural inclination to equate *more* with *better*, many coaches still train their athlete far too much, to the point that they are literally preventing results.

One very simple but badly misunderstood point must be corrected at the start. It is *impossible* to train *hard* and train a large amount at the same time. Coaches have no choice in the matter. They can have one or the other; they cannot have both. If they insist on a large amount of training, then they will be forced to reduce the intensity of training.

In some cases, an apparently large amount of training is required; it depends upon the sport, and upon the circumstances. A distance runner must train at running, more than a sprinter. No amount of 40-yard sprints will train a man properly for a 20-mile run. On the other hand, frequent practice of 20-mile runs will literally prevent a sprinter from improving his performance. In either case, there is a definite limit to the amount of training that either man can do while improving, or even maintaining his level of performance.

If the distance runner runs too much, his times will get worse instead of better and the same thing will happen to the sprinter. The sprinter must train with very high intensity. He must run as fast as possible for a short distance. The distance runner must *not* train in such fashion. If he attempts to run at a maximum level of intensity, it is extremely unlikely that he would last a full mile, much less 20 miles.

Therefore, the amount of training, and the intensity of training, must be directly related to the particular sport and they must be balanced in relation to each other. If the intensity is increased, then the amount of training must be reduced. A coach has no choice in the matter.

During the last few years, the trend has been in exactly the wrong direction in many sports, not in all sports, but in some sports. In a few sports, the results of overtraining are so obvious that it is impossible to miss the implications. In a few other sports, current training practices come fairly close to a practical balance between the intensity of training and the amount of training.

This balance is probably best in the sport of Olympic weight lifting, and we think we can demonstrate just why this is so. Weight lifting is one of the few sports in which the athlete is constantly more aware of his momentary ability, so a loss in strength is immediately obvious.

To lift a maximum weight, an athlete must perform at the highest possible intensity of effort, but if such maximum intensity is involved in every workout, then the workouts must be brief and infrequent. If not, then losses in strength will be produced instead of gains.

Olympic weight lifters have been forced to limit the amount of their training, and even if they fail to understand the exact cause and effect factors involved in this relationship between intensity of training and amount of training, they are at least aware of the practical implications.

As soon as the football season is finished, Mercury Morris starts to lose weight because he stops training. His normal body weight is considerably below his *conditioned* weight, so his weight drops when he stops training.

A muscle will not grow beyond its *normal* level unless such growth is stimulated by heavy exercise, but exercise is also required to maintain an existing high level of muscular mass. Therefore, a strong athlete will lose muscular size, and thus strength, if he stops training entirely.

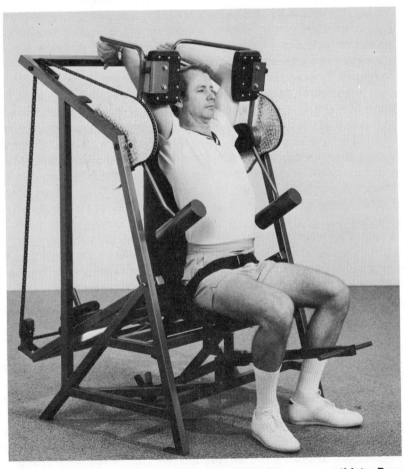

Do not expect exercise to turn an inferior athlete into a superathlete. Proper exercise will improve any athlete, and will improve some athletes to a degree that must literally be seen to be believed; but it cannot change bodily leverage, cannot improve reaction time and it cannot give an individual the judgment required by an outstanding athlete.

At least two factors will influence the rate at which such losses of strength will occur: 1) the difference between an athlete's *normal* weight and his *conditioned* weight; and 2) the length of time that an athlete has remained in good condition.

If a loss of body weight does not occur when training is stopped, then this is clear proof that fatty tissue is being added, and this is usually what happens in practice. Therefore, it is important to reduce the caloric intake in direct proportion to any reduction in the amount of training.

But it is equally important to avoid the trap of equating gains or losses to changes in body weight. It is easily possible to lose strength while gaining weight, or gain strength while losing weight. Progress must be measured on the basis of performance. If strength is increasing, then progress is being made regardless what may be happening to the body weight.

During the Colorado Experiment (detailed in later chapters), Casey Viator gained a total of 45.28 pounds in a period of 28 days, while reducing his starting level of body fat by 17.93 pounds. His actual gain in muscular mass (LBM) was 63.21 pounds. Conducted under strict laboratory conditions in the Physical Education Department at Colorado State University, this experiment clearly established the fact that very rapid increases in LBM can be produced while simultaneously reducing the level of fatty tissue.

Viator's results were produced by a total of 7 hours, 50.5 minutes of training within a period of exactly four weeks. He engaged in 14 workouts with an average time of 33.6 minutes per workout.

A large amount of training is neither necessary nor desirable. On the contrary, best results are usually produced by a very brief training schedule. Additional training may reduce the production of worthwhile results, and as an athlete grows stronger, his training program must be reduced.

The Best Type of Exercise

Just what is the best type of exercise? Properly conducted exercise is capable of producing a number of worthwhile results: 1) increased cardiovascular ability, or *condition*; 2) increased strength; 3) increased flexibility, or range of movement; 4) increased speed of movement; 5) increased muscular mass; 6) reduced fatty tissue; and 7) improved circulation. In addition, there are a large number of valuable results related to rehabilitation. Additionally, for reasons directly related to several of the previously mentioned factors, exercise can greatly reduce the chances of injury. Therefore, the choice of a type of exercise must be based upon the desired results.

In subsequent chapters in this book, we will cover every known type of exercise in great detail, step by step, point by point, in very simple terms.

In the meantime, a clear understanding must be established regarding certain basic points that are involved in any type of exercise. First, we must

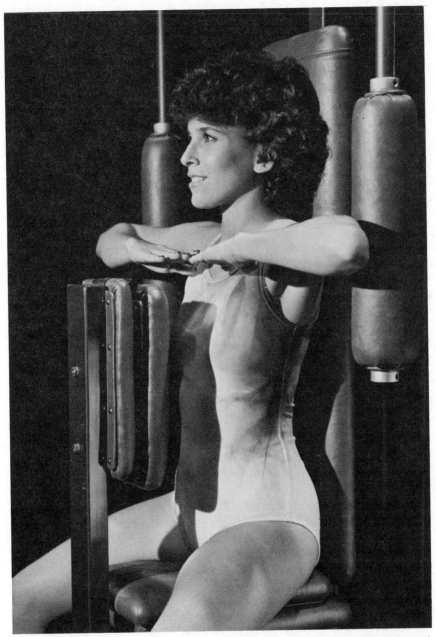

The best type of exercise is one that involves full-range movement, movement that starts from a fully extended, pre-stretched position and continues to a fully contracted position.

define the terms, and establish certain guidelines common to all types of exercise.

As mentioned previously, exercise can greatly reduce the chances of injury, but exercise is also capable of causing injury. The best type of exercise is the type that is most likely to prevent injury, and least likely to cause injury.

Jerky movements are directly responsible for a very high percentage of the injuries caused by exercise, and jerky movements are of little or no value for the purpose of developing strength. Exercises performed for the purpose of increasing strength should always be smooth. Sudden movements and *rapid accelerations* should be avoided.

In later chapters covering exact styles of performances, coaches will be informed that movement should be *as fast as possible in good form* in many exercises. But many people overlook the most important part of that sentence—*in good form*. They fail to realize that *as fast as possible* may be, in fact, quite slow. And in most cases, if the resistance is as heavy as it should be, *fastest possible movement* will be *quite slow.*

Sudden, jerky movements greatly increase the forces involved in exercise adding nothing to the exercise except the danger of injury. Therefore, it should be clearly understood right from the start that the form, or style of performance, is one of the most important factors in exercise. Without good form, there is little or nothing of value left in exercise.

Training for the sport of Olympic weight lifting requires the sudden movement of a weight, so in that case we have an exception but that is the only exception. All other athletes should avoid any sort of sudden movements during their strength-training programs.

Careful observation of proper form will produce best results in the way of increasing strength, and will go a long way in the direction of avoiding injury. For the purpose of *preventing* injury an exercise should involve stretching in the extended positions of the muscles being worked. Such stretching will also produce the benefit of greatly increased flexibility, which will in itself go a long way toward preventing injury.

The best type of exercise is one that involves full-range movement, movement that starts from a fully extended, pre-stretched position and continues to a fully contracted position. Anything less than a full-range movement will provide exercise for only part of a muscle, and will do little or nothing in the way of improving flexibility. Proper exercise, full-range exercise, will increase the range of movement of any athlete in any sport. It will increase his strength, increase his flexibility, increase his speed, and greatly reduce his chances of injury.

In a later chapter, we will cover the requirements for full-range exercise in great detail, but for the moment it is necessary only to be aware that full-range movement is an important factor in any type of exercise.

Finally, the best type of exercise for any purpose is progressive exercise.

Just what is progressive exercise? An exercise is progressive only if it involves constantly increasing work loads. The intensity of effort or the amount of training must be increased in proportion to increasing ability. As an athlete becomes stronger, he must work harder or more, but not both.

For the purpose of increasing cardiovascular ability the amount of training must be gradually increased up to a point, to a point far beyond the starting level. In this case, the intensity of training must *not* be raised too rapidly, nor too high. If an athlete is running for the purpose of improving his cardiovascular stamina, his results will be related almost directly to the amount of running within reasonable limits.

If he runs as fast as possible, thus involving maximum intensity, then it will simply be impossible to run as much as he should.

In general terms, there are two styles of training: 1) steady state or aerobic exercise; and 2) non-steady-state or anaerobic exercise.

A great deal of confusion exists in regard to these actually very simple points, confusion that we will attempt to eliminate, here and now.

A particular exercise can only be performed in one of two possible ways, either way, but not both ways at the same time. Walking at a pace that could be maintained for hours is steady-state exercise. Running at a pace that can be maintained only briefly is non-steady-state exercise.

This is a very important point that seems to be generally misunderstood. It is easily possible to arrange a training program in such a manner that an

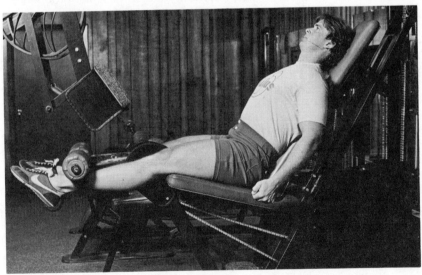

Without good form, there is little or nothing of value left in exercise.

athlete produces the potential benefits of both styles of training.

Steady-state training is necessary for cardiovascular benefits and non-steady-state exercise is required for meaningful strength increases. Both results can be produced from the same training program.

We stated previously that a *particular* exercise can only be performed in one of two possible ways, and that remains true. However, it is easily possible, and highly desirable, to arrange the training schedule in such a way that the muscles are being worked in a non-steady-state fashion while the *heart* and *lungs* are being worked in a steady-state fashion.

Strength training is usually performed in sports. A brief but very hard exercise is followed by a rest period. Conditioning training is usually performed at a much lower intensity, but for a much longer period of time, at a pace that will permit at least several minutes of steady exercise.

As a result of these widely practiced styles of training, many people have assumed that nothing else is possible. In fact, there is no reason why both styles cannot be combined into the same training schedule, at least in the training of active athletes, with Olympic weight-lifters again being the only important exception.

Steady-state training will *never* produce much in the way of meaningful strength increases, and non-steady-state training will do little or nothing for cardiovascular ability. However, a particular muscle can be worked to a point of momentary failure in a very brief period of time, in a non-steady-state fashion, and then another muscle can be worked immediately.

If the program is outlined properly, every major muscular group in the body can be worked in a non-steady-state fashion, while training the system as a whole in a steady-state fashion.

This is not merely a theory, it works. It works far better than any other style of training that we have ever tried, and we have tried everything we ever heard of that seemed to offer even the possibilty of worthwhile results, and quite a number of things that were obviously of non possible value.

Jerky movements are directly responsible for a very high percentage of the injuries caused by exercise, and jerky movements are of little or no value for the purpose of developing strength. Exercises performed for the purpose of increasing strength should always be smooth.

The Two Most Important Factors
in Exercise

The degree of results that can be produced by any form of exercise will always be limited by individual potential. In plain English, you cannot make a silk purse out of a sow's ear. But within the limits imposed by individual potential, the degree of results that will be produced will be determined largely by the quality of coaching to which an athlete is exposed.

The two most important factors in exercise may well be *individual potential and quality of coaching.*

This series of articles in this book can obviously do nothing towards improving the potential of athletes, but it can go a long way in the direction of giving coaches the information required for the intelligent coaching of athletes engaged in supplementary training for any sport.

Proper coaching consists of far more than an informed coaching staff. An active coaching staff is a factor of at least equal importance. Do not expect athletes to coach themselves; not many of them can, and even fewer will.

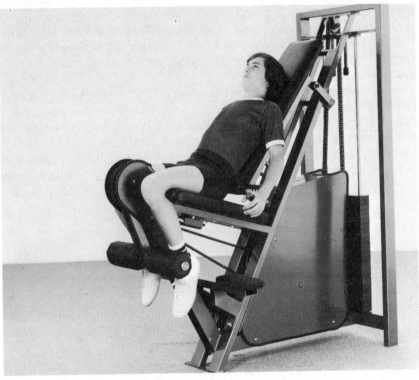

The degree of results that can be produced by any form of exercise will always be limited by individual potential.

This is particularly true when applied to the field of supplementary training, which many athletes tend to view as unnecessary drudgery. Most outstanding athletes will do a surprisingly good job of coaching themselves when they are engaged in an activity directly related to their sports specialty, but will also tend to view supplementary strength training as something of far less importance. They fail to realize that such training can well be the difference between success and failure in their chosen sport.

The actual cause and effect relationships involved in exercise are really quite simple, but widely misunderstood, even viewed with suspicion or doubt in areas where there is no room for any reasonable doubt.

In this series of chapters, we will attempt to remove those doubts in the only way that such doubts can be removed, by providing plain-language information based upon established facts.

Physiology simply means the physics of biology or biological physics. However, this seems to have been largely forgotten or overlooked.

Certain basic laws of physics apply with equal validity in all situations, which means that the human body and the engine of an automobile have a great deal in common. Clearly understanding the function of one will take a coach a long way in the direction of understanding the function of the other.

At this point in time nobody seriously claims to know exactly *why* a muscle responds to exercise by growing stronger. But we do know how to produce this result.

Practical experience has clearly and repeatedly established the fact that proper exercise is capable of producing literally enormous increases in muscular strength. And practical experience has also established the fact that no amount of low-intensity exercise will produce the results that come from an actually small amount of high-intensity training. We can conjecture to our heart's content about exactly why this is so, but in the meantime we can also make good, practical application of the fact that it is so.

4
Progressive Exercise

By Arthur Jones

Below a certain threshold of intensity, exercise will do little or nothing in the way of increasing strength. But if the intensity is high enough, a very brief program of exercise will produce rapid increases in strength if training is truly progressive.

We have already mentioned three factors that have never been satisfactorily defined—*intensity, strength, and progressive.* Until and unless we reach an understanding of those terms, no meaningful discussion of exercise is possible. We do not suggest that our definitions are the only possible defintions, but we do feel that they are satisfactory for our purposes here.

Intensity, as we will use the term, means *muscular intensity.* Maximum intensity is involved only when a muscle is pulling as hard as momentarily possible, producing as much force as it is capable of producing at that moment. A moment's consideration thus makes it obvious that intensity cannot be determined by measuring output. The following example should make this clear.

If a 100-pound barbell is resting on a platform scale, the weight will produce a *downwards* force of 100 pounds and the scale will register 100 pounds. But if the trainee grasps the barbell and exerts a force of 50 pounds in an *upwards* direction, then the scale will register only 50 pounds. Note carefully that the barbell will not move. If the trainee were pulling as hard as momentarily possible, then the intensity would be maximum. But if he were not pulling as hard as possible, then it is probably impossible to measure the intensity that was involved. In both cases we were accurately measuring the output, but intensity was determined only when it was maximum.

47

During a normal set of 10 repetitions with a barbell, the level of intensity varies from repetition to repetition, constantly increases, and is maximum only during the final repetition, and then only if the final repetition leads to a point of momentary failure. If it was possible to perform an eleventh repetition, then the intensity never reached a maximum level. Maximum intensity is produced only if an exercise is carried to a point where another repetition is momentarily impossible. So we can measure maximum intensity, but only under certain circumstances.

During the first repetition of a set of 10 repetitions, the intensity is low, even though the output is actually higher during the first repetition than it is during the final repetition. An example follows.

If a trainee curls a 100-pound barbell in a strict manner, performing 10 repetitions and failing during an attempt to perform an eleventh repetition, then the output is high and the intensity is low during the first repetition, and the output is low and the intensity is high during the tenth repetition. During the first repetition the trainee was momentarily capable of doing more, and could have lifted more weight than he was lifting. The weight was lifted, thus the output was high, but it was lifted easily, so the intensity was low. During the tenth repetition the trainee was not momentarily capable of doing more. If the weight had been any heavier, then he could not have lifted it. So again the weight was lifted, but it was lifted slower, thus the output was lower than it was during the first repetition, and since the trainee was working as hard as possible, the intensity was high.

It should now be obvious that intensity is a relative situation depending upon momentary ability, varying moment by moment, and not directly related to output. If the trainee could have done more, but did not, then the intensity was low. But the intensity is maximum if he is doing all he can at the moment regardless of how much or how little output is actually involved.

It should also be mentioned that the production of force is related to output, and can be measured, but a high level of force is not required for high intensity. In fact, if exercises are performed properly, then the maximum intensity repetitions will actually involve less force. It is easily possible and very desirable to have high intensity and low force at the same time. A failure to understand this simple point has led to a ridiculous situation that is very commonly encountered in exercise programs.

Many, perhaps most, trainees avoid the final two or three repetitions in a set under the totally mistaken belief that they are thus avoiding the most *dangerous* repetitions. In fact, the final repetitions are actually the safest, because the output is lower, the production of force is lower. During the final repetition the trainee is imposing less pulling force on his muscular attachments than he was during the first few repetitions.

In practice, thousands of trainees avoid the most productive repetitions

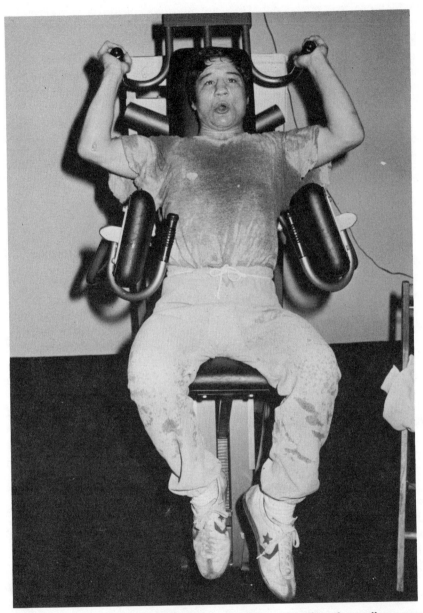

It should be obvious that intensity is a relative situation depending upon momentary ability, varying moment by moment, and not directly related to output. If the trainee could have done more, but did not, then the intensity was low. But the intensity is maximum if he is doing all he can at the moment regardless of how much or how little output is actually involved.

under the false impression that they are thus avoiding the *dangerous* repetitions. But they have already performed the most dangerous repetitions, the first few repetitions, and are actually skipping the safest repetitions. As a direct consequence, most trainees produce results that are far below optimum results, because a very high percentage of the strength increases produced by exercise is a direct result of high intensity, which is involved only in the final two or three repetitions.

Several years of exercise that is stopped three repetitions short of a point of momentary failure will not produce results equal to those that can be produced in a matter of a few weeks by an otherwise exactly similar training program that is carried to a point of momentary failure.

The final two or three repetitions are merely *preparation* and do little or nothing in the way of increasing strength. These repetitions are of little value because the intensity is low. The final repetitions are productive because the intensity is high.

Since the facts in this case, simple and undeniable though they are, run directly contrary to very widespread belief, it will be a long time before this point is understood and accepted by a high percentage of trainees or coaches. In the meantime, most strength programs will consist primarily of wasted effort. Millions of man-hours of training and billions of foot-pounds of effort will be devoted to programs that produce little if anything of value.

Gains in strength will come slowly, if at all. Trainees will lose interest from a lack of progress, and coaches will look elsewhere in search of some *secret* to more rapid strength increases. Many trainees (and coaches) will make the old mistake of equating more with better. When progress is less than expected, they will increase the *amount* of training, under the mistake of equating more with better. When progress is less than expected, they will increase the *amount* of training, under the mistaken belief that training more means training harder. In fact, all that is required is an increase in the intensity of exercise.

Most trainees who do stick to a strength program for a long period of time eventually fall into a pattern of training where their workouts are about as productive as walking cross-country on a treadmill. The intensity of their workouts is seldom if ever high enough to stimulate strength increases, but the *amount* of training is so high that they remain in a constantly run-down condition.

Under such circumstances, growth is seldom stimulated but will be slow in all cases, and impossible in many cases, because the recovery ability will be constantly forced to work as hard as possible merely to replace the large amount of energy that is required, leaving nothing as a reserve for growth.

It must be clearly understood that high-intensity training and a *large amount* of training are mutually exclusive factors. A trainee can have one or

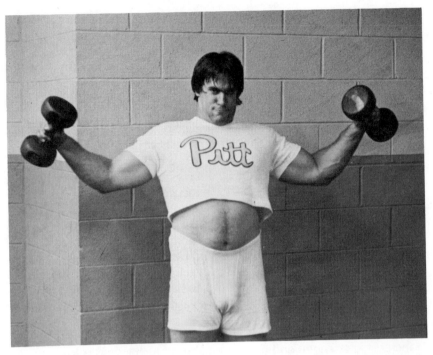

It must be clearly understood that high-intensity training and a large amount of training are mutually exclusive factors.

the other, but not both. If he doubles the intensity of training, then he must reduce the amount of training by more than 80 percent in order to compensate for the increased intensity. If not, then he will produce losses in strength instead of gains.

Since it is very difficult to measure an intensity level less than maximum, how do we prove that point? How can we test such a theory? Very easily. A trainee should determine just how much weight he can curl for ten repetitions in perfect form with an eleventh repetition being impossible.

Let us assume this weight turns out to be 100 poounds. Then use exactly half as much weight, 50 pounds, and perform 20 sets of curls with this reduced weight during each of three weekly training sessions. After six months of such training, with no other training of any kind, the trainee should test his ability with 100 pounds again and not be surprised if he is actually weaker than he was at the start. He probably will not be weaker, but he will certainly be a little, if any, stronger. A large *amount* of low-intensity exercise did very little for increasing strength, probably nothing, and may even have produced losses.

Now double the weight, go back to the 100 pounds and perform 20 sets of as many repetitions as possible with 100 pounds. Perform as many repetitions as possible in each set, because the trainee will not be capable of performing 10 repetitions in each of 20 sets during the same workout. Again follow a program of three weekly workouts, 20 sets of curls in each workout, and no other exercise. Watch what happens, and the trainee should not be surprised by the fact that he will lose strength rapidly, and grow steadily weaker. At least he would if such a comparison was made using exercises for all of the major muscular structures in the body.

Recovery ability is an *overall* thing. It is related to the system as a whole. An individual muscle (such as the biceps) is capable of very rapid recovery from an enormous amount of work if the recovery ability of the system is not depleted.

Testing one muscle in isolation is really not a good test, because one small muscle can perform a great deal of work without imposing much strain on the recovery ability. A better test would involve larger muscles, for example an exercise such as the squat. But for actually valid results, a test should involve a variety of exercises, at least 8 basic exercises, covering all of the major muscular structures. When such a valid test is conducted, the results can be accurately predicted in advance.

A large amount of low-intensity exercise will do little or nothing in the way of increasing strength, and a large amount of high-intensity exercise will produce losses in strength. Instead, if the trainee reduced the number of sets to only 1 or 2, instead of 20, and doubled the weight used during the large amount of low-intensity exercise, then rapid and steady strength increases would be produced as long as the intensity was as high as momentarily possible during each set, and as long as each set was continued to a point of failure. In such a case, he would be performing only 20 percent as much exercise insofar as *amount* of exercise is concerned—10 percent as many sets, but twice as much weight. Obviously, then the *amount* of exercise was reduced 80 percent by comparison to the low-intensity exercise program. Yet the results would be much better.

In spite of all of the clear evidence, most trainees still persist in doing more when they should be working less, but working harder. To produce good results from exercise, trainees must work harder, and if they work harder, then they must work less.

Strength

Strength has never been properly defined, but until we agree on an acceptable meaning, no reasonable discussion of strength training (or exercise) is possible. First, we think it is necessary to realize that the strength of one man can never be fairly compared to that of another. Far too many variables are involved to permit such a comparison.

How far was the weight lifted? Did each man lift it an equal distance? If not, then the comparison was invalid. How fast was the weight lifted? Was the speed of movement exactly the same in both cases? If not, then the production of *power* was different even if the weight was the same in both cases, and even if the distance of movement was also equal.

What about skill? Was that exactly equal? Two men will never be exactly equal. They will always be unequal in too many ways to permit accurate strength comparisons.

It should also be noted from the start that it is not necessary to compare a man's strength to that of another man. For our purposes, we need compare a man only to himself at another point in time.

Exercise performed for the purpose of increasing strength is productive if a man's strength is increasing, increasing in relation to his strength at an earlier point in time. It is easily possible to greatly increase a man's *apparent strength* or his *demonstratable strength* by merely teaching him a better style of lifting while doing absolutely nothing in the way of increasing his actual strength.

We think *actual strength increases* should only be measured by comparing performances that are exactly the same in all respects except the amount of weight involved. We also feel that such comparisons should involve only movements that are performed at a fairly slow speed, and in perfect form.

We do not believe in the validity of maximum, single-attempt lifts. For example, a man might bench press 200 pounds, and then be unable to perform a second repetition with the same weight. Later, he might use 300 pounds and again fail when trying a second repetition with the same weight.

Is he thus 50 percent stronger? Perhaps, but perhaps not. He might be more than 50 percent stronger, or less than 50 percent stronger. During the first test, he might have been capable of using 210 pounds, if he had tried it instead of the 200. During the second test, he might have been capable of 310, but having reduced his strength by the lift with 300, he was then unable to demonstrate his actual level of strength on that day.

Such comparisons of maximum-attempt lifts are only *fairly accurate* at best and usually, in practice, fall far short of real accuracy of measurement.

A much better comparison of strength, we feel, is based on an ability to perform several repetitions, a reasonable number from about 6 to 12, as long as the number is always the same, and as long as each set leads to a point of failure.

The problem here stems from the fact that sets carried to a point of failure do not always result in the same number of repetitions, and how can 8 repetitions with 200 pounds be compared reasonably to 11 repetitions with 240 pounds?

Such a comparison cannot be made beyond noting that the second per-formance indicated a *stronger* performance. This is not the perfect system of measuring strength, but it is the best one we have found in more than 30 years of looking.

In practice, using the system of strength measurement means that com-parisons cannot be made on a day-by-day basis, except in general terms, which, for our purposes, is actually the best method of charting strength in-creases. While we will not always know the exact strength level at a particu-lar point in time, we will be instantly aware of changes in strength, either in-creases or losses.

For example, if a trainee performs 7 repetitions with 200 pounds on Mon-day, and then 8 with 200 on Wednesday, he is obviously stronger, even though we do not know exactly how much stronger. But if he does 7 with 200 on Monday, and then only 6 on Wednesday, then he is weaker and is losing strength. For all practical purposes, a trainee will produce sets that do result in exactly the same number of repetitions often enough to give a very accu-rate chart of his progress.

We can hear the howls of protest from some quarters—"But that is not measuring strength, that is endurance." We might as well settle that point here and now, or at least try to settle it, being well aware in advance that many people will never accept the facts in the matter—having misun-derstood the relationship between *strength* and *endurance* for too many years.

Some people will die with the firm belief that *strength* is one thing and that *endurance* is something else. In fact, they are one and the same thing, exactly the same thing, and if one is measured accurately, then the other is obvious, or should be.

This brings us to the definition of *endurance*. Keep it clearly in mind that we mean *muscular endurance*. We are not talking about cardiovascular ability, or cardiopulmonary ability. We are not talking about the ability of the heart or lungs. We are talking about the ability of the muscles to perform several consecutive repetitions repeatedly with a weight that could be lifted for one maximum attempt repetition.

As long as the weight and the speed of performance are such that a trainee reaches a point of failure after 6 to 12 repetitions, then he is testing *strength* as well as *endurance*. If the weight is so light that the number of repetitions becomes very high, then other factors come into play, and the test is no longer valid for testing either strength or endurance of the muscle itself. Such high repetition, low-resistance exercises will not do much in the way of building strength in any case, so we need not concern ourselves with them.

A great deal of confusion on this point probably arises from attempts to

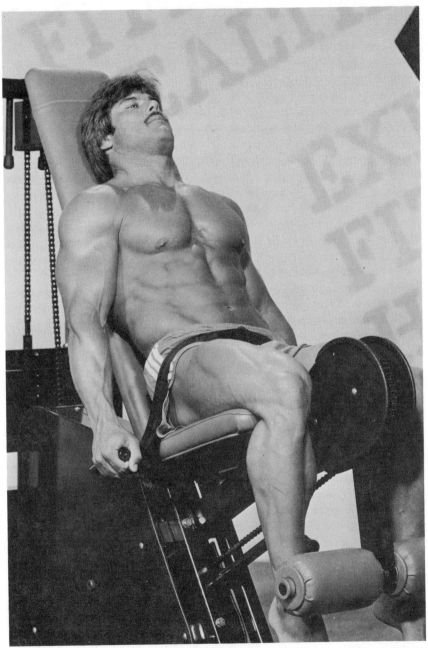

...In fact, instructions for producing maximum results from exercise can be reduced to four words, train hard, train briefly.

compare one man's strength to another man's endurance, which simply cannot be done with anything approaching accuracy. If we restrict our attempts to measure strength, or endurance, to comparisons between two or more different performances by the same man, we will avoid most of the problems leading to misunderstanding.

What frequently happens is something like the following. On a particular date, during the same workout, a man bench presses 300 pounds for one maximum-attempt repetition, and performs 10 repetitions with 250 pounds, failing when he attempts an eleventh repetition. Then he stops training for a period of several weeks, during which period of time his strength declines.

Upon starting to train again, he knows he cannot duplicate the 300-pound lift so he does not attempt it. He guesses that perhaps his strength has declined by 10 percent, reduces the bar by that percentage, takes 270 pounds for his maximum attempt, and makes it about as easily as he previously lifted the 300 pounds. He is correct in his impression that his strength had declined by 10 percent. Then he makes a mistake that leads to a false conclusion. He takes 250 pounds to test his endurance, and is able to perform only 4 repetitions, instead of the 10 he did previously.

He wrongly assumes from this result that his *endurance* has declined by 60 percent while his *strength* went down only 10 percent. Thus he thinks his endurance dropped much more than his strength, but he thinks wrong. The test was invalid.

To be valid, he would have to test his *endurance* with 225 pounds. He would have to reduce the endurance test weight by exactly the same percentage that he reduced the strength test weight, not reduce it by the same amount, but by the same percentage. If he did so, then he would have been able to perform 10 repetitions, exactly the same number that he did previously with the heavier weight.

It would then be obvious that his strength and endurance declined in exact proportion to each other. They would go up and down together, maintaining a definite relationship.

If at a particular point in time, a trainee can bench press 200 pounds ten times and can lift 240 pounds once, then the ability to perform two repetitions at a later point in time with 400 pounds will indicate that the individual has the strength to lift 480 pounds once. Thus, if he doubles his *endurance* he has also doubled his *strength* to the extent that style and confidence do not become involved, and to the extent that strength means the ability of a muscle to produce force.

Failing to understand this point, simple and undeniable as it actually is, or failing to agree with the explanation which we consider to be perfectly clear and beyond dispute, some readers will be *turned off* by anything else we have to say. But we think it only fair to remind these readers that the only rational reason for reading any of this is an attempt to learn something. If, however, they are merely looking for additional confirmation of firmly-held beliefs, then we would strongly advise them to skip the rest of our writing. Because careful research and simple logic have already taught us that most of the current beliefs on the subject of exercise are without basis in fact, and experience has taught us that many people are apparently unwilling to change their beliefs, regardless of the evidence that is presented.

We are well aware in advance that even mention of *controversial* subjects such as the relationship between strength and endurance will close the minds of many readers, we also know that the entire field of exercise will remain firm in the presently existing *dark ages* until and unless the light of logic is turned on the subject.

Therefore, in later chapters, I will clearly outline the practical *how to do it* and *what results to expect* from what type of programs. I will also outline the requirements that are required for producing the maximum degree of results from exercise at this point in time, the state of the art being what it is, with the knowledge that presently exists.

In fact, instructions for producing maximum results from exercise can be reduced to four words: *train hard, train briefly.*

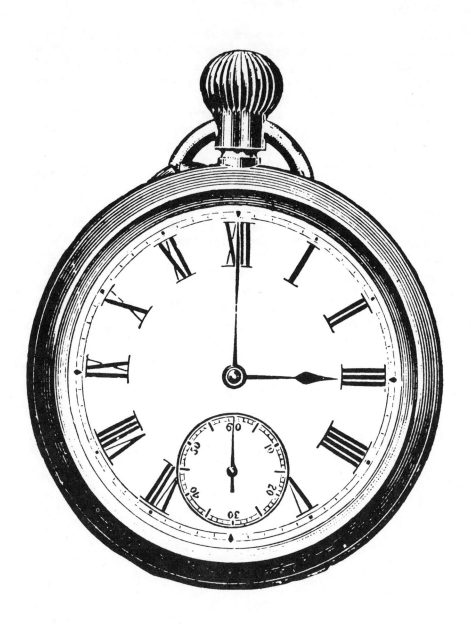

5
Time As a Factor in Exercise

By Arthur Jones

Time is a factor in almost everything...a very important factor in exercise for a number of reasons. Many of the problems in exercise are directly related to time.

About thirty years ago, somebody said..."Instead of trying to find out just how much exercise you can stand, we should be trying to determine how little exercise we really need."

Yet, thirty years later, we still find most people training far too much...and make no mistake on this point, the most common mistake in exercise today is gross overtraining, far too much exercise.

This simply proves that one of the time factors in exercise is widely misunderstood...but so are the others misunderstood and thus incorrectly applied; the result being that most of the time devoted to exercise is wasted, and a large part of the time is actually counterproductive.

Properly applied, any and all time devoted to exercise should be productive...and it can be, but seldom is. In very simple terms, this means that every minute devoted to exercise should produce a certain result, a measurable result; if not, then the time is wasted...or worse, may actually produce a loss in functional ability rather than an increase.

Proper exercise is capable of producing steady and rapid increases in functional ability...greater strength, increased flexibility, improved cardiovascular condition, faster speed of movement, and other very worthwhile benefits. And, contrary to popular opinion, it does not take years to produce such benefits...or it should not, it need not; but in practice it usually does...it usually does because most people have no clear understanding of the really simple cause and effect relationships involved in exercise.

Time As a Factor in Exercise

Opinions? Oh, yes...they certainly have opinions and strong beliefs; but facts and opinions seldom have much if anything in common. As a result, we see thousands of people putting their opinions into practice...then spending years in an attempt to produce a result that could have been produced in a matter of weeks.

Exercise is performed for only one of two possible reasons...one, for the purpose of stimulating a physical change...or, two, for the purpose of preventing a physical change.

On the one hand, exercise is performed in an attempt to prevent a loss in one of these same areas of functional ability. So exercise is thus intended either to stimulate change or to prevent change.

But please note that exercise does not produce a change of any kind...no worthwhile change at least. Any actual change that is produced by exercise will almost certainly be an injury of some sort. Changes that result from exercise are actually produced by the body itself...all that exercise can do is stimulate the body change.

So, the real purpose of exercise is stimulation...and properly applied exercise will provide growth stimulation of one kind or another. And, once stimulated, the healthy body will change in a worthwhile manner.

Many hundreds of examples of very rapid growth clearly prove that the body is certainly capable of producing rapid and large-scale increases in muscular size, strength, flexibility, and cardiovascular condition...and remember, it is the body that produces such changes, not exercise.

All that exercise does is stimulate change, it does not produce change.

So, if the body is capable of producing a rapid rate of change, which it is, and if the actual changes occur very slowly...then obviously something is wrong. Something is wrong with the exercise.

And, it should be clearly understood...if the stimulation is proper, then very little stimulation is required. Whereas, if the stimulation is incorrect, then no amount of improper stimulation will produce a worthwhile result.

You might compare exercise and growth to a stick of dynamite and a hammer. If you hit a stick of dynamite lightly with a hammer, nothing will happen. It makes no difference how many times you hit it, as long as the blows are light...because a light blow will not stimulate an explosion, and several light blows are not equal to one heavy blow.

But, if you hit it hard, then only one blow is required. Below a certain level of force, no stimulation is produced...but above a certain level of force, the required stimulation is provided and an explosion will result.

Much the same sort of situation exists in exercise...light exercise will not provide the stimulation required for change; so heavy exercise is an absolute requirement for the stimulation of physical improvement...but large amounts of such stimulation are neither necessary nor desirable. In effect, it takes only one hard blow with the hammer to set off the explosion.

It takes only one properly placed shot to kill a rabbit, or an elephant...additional shots will serve no purpose except unnecessary destruction of the meat. And the same thing is true in exercise; having properly stimulated growth, then you must leave the body alone and permit it to respond to the stimulation...and that takes time. The stimulation of growth can occur almost instantly, but the growth that occurs as a result of such stimulation cannot occur instantly...instead, it takes time, a minimum of two days and sometimes longer.

So exercise should not be repeated too frequently...and in practice this means that you should not perform more than three workouts within a period of a week. Daily training is neither necessary nor desirable...additional workouts will not produce better results. On the contrary, four weekly workouts will produce less results than three weekly workouts...five weekly workouts will produce very little in the way of worthwhile results...and six or seven weekly workouts may well produce an actual loss in functional ability. So, in the case of exercise at least, more is certainly not better.

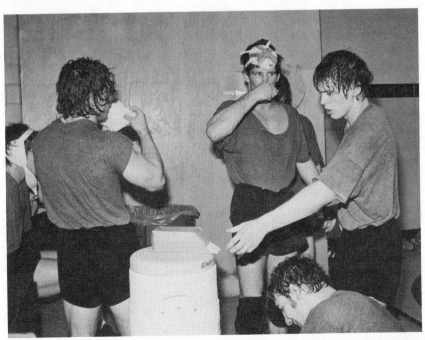

A certain period of rest is required between hard workouts, but this rest period should be neither too short nor too long; in general, you should permit at least forty-eight hours of rest between hard workouts, but not more than ninety-six hours.

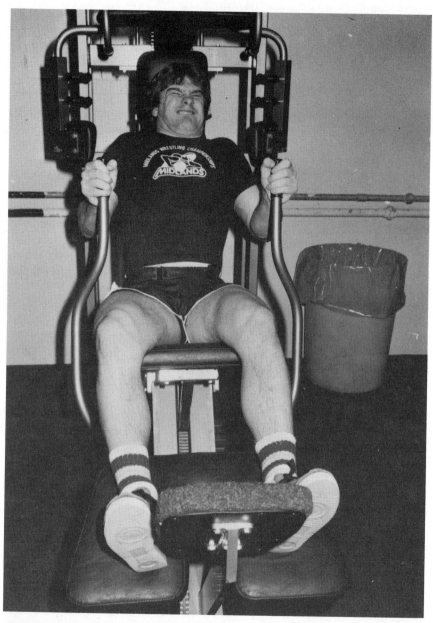

Do not continue an exercise to the point where it becomes necessary to change the style of performance in order to continue...doing so will result in throwing the weight instead of lifting it, and this is neither necessary nor desirable.

Proper frequency of workouts thus becomes the first rule involving the time factor in exercise...train often enough, but not too often; in practice this means at least two weekly workouts, but not more than three.

Why a minimum of two weekly workouts...and why a maximum of three weekly workouts?

Because, if you train less than twice a week, the resulting period between workouts will be too long...and if you train more than three times a week, then the resting period between workouts will be too short. A certain period of rest is required between hard workouts, but this rest period should be neither too short nor too long; in general, you should permit at least forty-eight hours of rest between hard workouts, but not more than ninety-six hours.

Less than forty-eight hours between hard workouts will not allow enough time for full recovery...more than ninety-six hours is too long.

On a three workout per week schedule, Monday, Wednesday, Friday for example, you are permitting forty-eight hours of rest between Monday and Wednesday workouts, and between the Wednesday and Friday work-outs...and seventy-two hours of rest between the Friday and Monday work-outs. In most cases, this is the best schedule.

But please note that I said hard workouts...which is not meant to imply that no activity of any kind should occur during the rest period between hard workouts. Normal or even medium level activity will have no adverse ef-fect...but do avoid any really high-intensity activity between workouts. In ef-fect, train for strength three times weekly, and train very hard but very briefly...then work on your skill during the off-days between workouts.

Regardless of your condition, you cannot fully recover from a hard work-out in less than forty-eight hours, but light or medium activity during the rest period will not prevent or delay your recovery.

At the start of training you will have little or no desire to train hard more than three times weekly...but later, as your strength and condition improve, there will be a strong temptation to train more often; but do not, since train-ing too often is one of the worst mistakes you can make. If your progress is less than you hoped for, then chances are that you are training too much rather than too little...training more is almost never the answer. Believe it or not, training too little is far better than training too much; and if you are devot-ing more than two hours weekly strength training, then you are training too much.

That is right, two hours a week are too much...yet, in practice, we see thousands of people training three or four hours a day. But it should be clearly understood that such people are not training that much and training hard...they are training a lot, but they are not training very hard. Three hours of actual hard training during one workout would put a well-conditioned gorilla into the hospital...and a week of such daily workouts would put him into a grave. The idea is to stimulate growth, not to kill yourself...and it takes very little hard training to produce maximum growth stimulation. Remember, training merely stimulates growth; it does not produce growth.

Which brings us to the next time-related factor in exercise, the length of time that should be devoted to each workout. Which point is subject to misunderstanding...and which point is largely determined by the purpose of the training.

If the training is performed only for the purpose of increasing strength, then any reasonable length of time can be devoted to the workout without ill effect upon the production of results...although, even in this case, the workout should not require more than an hour.

However, if the training is performed for the two purposes of increasing strength and improving cardiovascular condition, as it should be, then the training time should be shorter.

Exactly how much shorter? Well, this is where the misunderstanding may enter the picture; the workout should be as brief as possible without compromising the strength building aspects...which qualifications I will not attempt to explain.

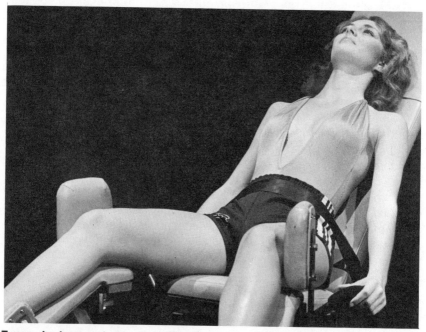

Every single exercise in the entire workout must be performed in the same manner...each exercise must be carried as far as possible to squeeze out one more repetition in good form.

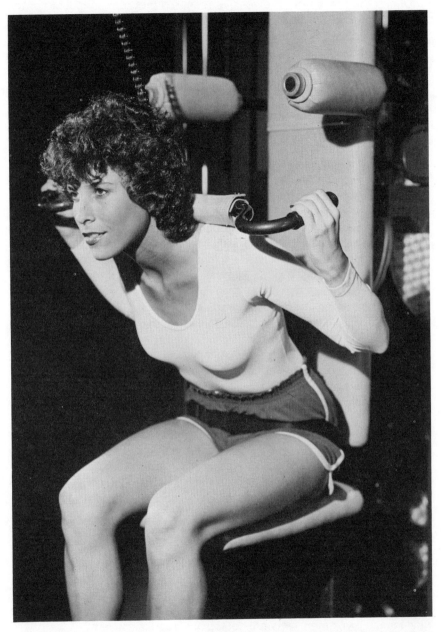

Properly performed exercise is capable of producing far better results than most people even suspect...so, since you are spending the time and making the investment, why not get the best results you can?

Time As a Factor in Exercise

During the course of an extensive research program conducted at the United States Military Academy, West Point in April and May of 1975, a large group of varsity football players increased their strength an average of nearly 60 percent within a period of only six weeks. As a result of only seventeen brief workouts that averaged less than thirty minutes each, a total of less than eight hours of training time, almost unbelievable results were obtained.

These subjects performed only one set of approximately twelve exercises in every workout, and their speed of movement was fairly slow; yet their average level of improvement was several times as great as any results ever shown by anybody else in any other research program; literally several hundred percent better...a level of improvement that was previously considered impossible, and is impossible with any other type or style of training.

No injuries were caused during the program, and several subjects who started the program suffering from previously injured hamstring muscles, finished the program with no remaining traces of injury...having totally recovered from their previous injuries and having greatly increased the strength of their hamstrings as well as all other major muscular structures in the body.

In addition to the enormous average strength increases, these subjects also improved their cardiovascular condition to the point that they reduced their average time for the two mile run by eighty-eight seconds...and they also improved their flexibility from ten to twenty times as much as a control group of other football players who were trained in a conventional fashion.

Such results are not accidental, and such results cannot be produced in any other fashion...but it should also be clearly understood that such results probably cannot be produced without supervision; most subjects either cannot or will not push themselves to the point required for best results, so supervision is of great importance, and this is true regardless of the equipment being used.

But you certainly would not consider sending your squad out to practice without supervision, so why should you expect them to be able to train properly without supervision.

Supervision does not produce results, but it should assure a proper style of performance...and remember, a proper style of performance is frequently the only difference between very good results and no results at all. This is equally true in exercise or anything else.

Properly performed exercise is capable of producing far better results than most people even suspect...so, since you are spending the time and making the investment, why not get the best results you can?

6
Avoiding and Preventing Injuries

By Arthur Jones

Exercise should help to avoid injury...not cause injury. But, it can do either. It can strengthen the muscles and joints of an athlete to such an extent that the possibility of a directly sports-connected injury is greatly reduced. Or...if improperly performed, it can cause injury that might never have occurred on the playing field.

Exercise can cause *injury* in at least two different ways...1) an athlete may injure himself while performing an exercise, an injury that is a direct result of exercise...or 2) an athlete may hurt himself on the field as an *indirect* result of exercise.

Strength increases are stimulated by high intensity of work, and only by high intensity of work...a muscle must be worked to, or very near, a point of momentary failure. In practice it appears that approximately eight to twelve repetitions should be used for upperbody exercises and about twenty repetitions for lowerbody exercises...but regardless of the actual number of repetitions performed, the exercise must be continued to a point where it is momentarily impossible to perform another repetition in good form.

In effect, if you could have done twelve repetitions but stopped after only ten, then that exercise was probably wasted...little or no growth stimulation will be produced.

Do not continue an exercise to the point where it becomes necessary to change the style of performance in order to continue...doing so will result in throwing the weight instead of lifting it. This is neither necessary nor desirable, but dangerous.

Do continue for as many repetitions as you can possibly manage in good form...do not terminate the exercise simply because the movements become very hard, or because the muscles start to ache; strength building exercise literally must be hard, and if it is properly performed it will make the muscles ache.

In a set of twelve repetitions leading to a point of failure after the twelfth repetition, the first ten repetitions are largely preparation...most, perhaps all, of the actual growth stimulation is produced by the final two very hard repetitions. So, if you stop one or two repetitions short of a point of actual momentary muscular failure, then a very large part, perhaps all, of the benefit will be missed.

Every single exercise in the entire workout must be performed in this same manner...each exercise must be carried as far as possible in good form. Do not terminate any exercise if it is possible to squeeze out one more repetition in good form.

Then...when one exercise is properly completed, move on to the next exercise as soon as possible; but not too quickly...not so quickly that your breathing or pulse rate acts as a limiting factor.

If you move on to the next exercise too quickly, then you may become lightheaded...or you may even become nauseated. So, you must permit a short breathing space between exercises...at least at the start of actual heavy training.

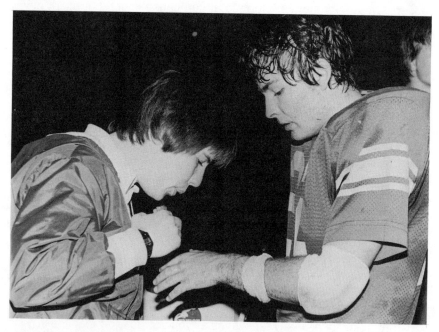

Exercise should help to avoid injury...not cause injury.

At first, you may require about two minutes of rest between exercises; but, as time passes, you should gradually reduce the rest period between exercises...and, eventually, you should be able to go through a full workout with little or no rest between exercises. It may require two months of really hard training before you reach a condition where you can go through a full workout almost nonstop, moving immediately from one exercise to the next.

But do not rush it too much...if you do, then you will be unable to work the muscles as hard as they really require for best results. And do not permit the workouts to degenerate into a race against the clock; your total time for a workout should gradually decrease, and it will...but the important thing is to be very sure that the muscles are worked properly, but they will not be if you rush through the workout too fast.

Try to treat each exercise as a thing unto itself, as if each exercise were the complete workout; try not to think about what has happened before or what is to follow...if you hold back in anticipation of the next exercise, then you are defeating the purpose.

This brings us to the next time-related factor, the speed of movement during the exercises. This point, at the moment, is a point of enormous controversy...with some people saying train as fast as possible, and others saying almost the opposite. So just what is the best speed of movement? Well, quite frankly, nobody knows...although some people would have you believe that they do know.

But I can tell you what we have learned from our own experience; we have found that a fairly slow speed of movement produces far better results than a fast speed of movement...much, much better results.

I can also tell you, and I can prove, that a fast speed of movement during exercise does the following: it jerks the muscles violently during the first few degrees of movement...after which point the weight is moving so fast that the muscles literally are not involved in the rest of the movement. The result being that a dangerous yank is imposed on the muscles at the start of the movement and then absolutely nothing is accomplished during most of the movement. In such cases you are throwing the weight, not lifting it...and such a style of training will produce nothing but injuiries.

Yet, in practice, that is exactly how many people train...which probably explains why it takes them years to produce a degree of results that could have been produced in an equal number of weeks; and it certainly explains why people who practice such a style of training eventually injure themselves seriously.

And...do not be confused by the current crop of double-talk about fast-twitch and slow-twitch muscle fibers; which is another subject that absolutely nothing is known about at this point in time...although, again, this is a subject where some people would like to mislead you into believing that they do know quite a lot about the subject. We have conducted at least ten times as much research in the field of strength training as everybody else in the exercise business combined...and this is a very conservative statement. At the moment we are building the largest and best equipped human performance center in the world, and this is in preparation for extremely large-scale research projects involving literally thousands of subjects...and we are in close, direct communications with the leading research scientists now involved in a study of different muscle-fiber types.

If and when we do learn something of value regarding different muscle types, then we will publish the information.,..and in the meantime, every single one of the articles on this subject that has come to my attention in popular journals consisted of pure hogwash and gross misquotes taken entirely out of context.

In closing this point, let me repeat that I do not personally know anything on this subject that has the slightest relationship to a practical application in exercise...and neither does anybody else.

As recently as four years ago, we used a very fast speed of movement in exercise...but since then we have learned better, and I am certainly not ashamed to admit my past mistakes...and now we produce better results in six weeks than we used to produce in six months.

A fast speed of movement during exercise does the following: it jerks the muscles violently during the first few degrees of movement...after which point the weight is moving so fast that the muscles literally are not involved in the rest of the movement. The result being that a dangerous yank is imposed on the muscles at the start of the movement then absolutely nothing is accomplished during most of the movement. In such cases you are throwing the weight not lifting it...and such a style of training will produce nothing but injuries.

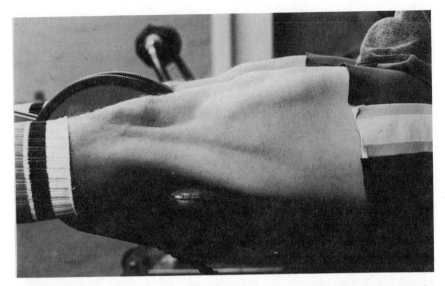

In fact, simple common sense also makes it obvious that a stronger man is less likely to be injured in any given situation...and that a more flexible man is also less prone to injury.

Injury that is directly caused by exercise will usually be obvious, and the coach will normally be aware of such an accident when it happens and will thus know where to place the blame. But *indirect* injury may not be so easy to recognize, since it will not result from a simple cause and effect type of situation that makes itself known immediately.

For example, if an athlete pulls a thigh muscle while performing squats in the gymnasium, the coach will know exactly where to place the blame. But if, instead, he pulls a hamstring on the field...the coach might not realize that the injury was an *indirect* result of exercise. And it might not be...*but it could be.*

If an exercise program results in a disproportionate muscular development in antagonistic muscles, then it is almost asking for trouble. For example, if an athlete develops great strength in the muscles of the frontal thigh while doing little or nothing to increase the strength of the rear of the thigh, then he may actually cause an injury. This injury would probably occur on the field, and probably would not be blamed on exercise.

Unfortunately, since the blame for such indirectly caused injury is seldom placed where it belongs, it is utterly impossible to estimate the number of such injuries with any reasonable degree of accuracy...but, I am personally convinced that the number would be quite high.

Thus, the *known* injuries from exercise, when added to the *unknown*, equal a high but unsuspected total.

Balanced against the unknown total, we have only another *unknown* factor in the way of compensation; since, obviously, it is also impossible to estimate the number of injuries that were *prevented* by exercise. After all, who can even guess just how many injuries *might have happened.*

Therefore, on the surface it may well appear that exercise merely causes injuries...while offering nothing in the way of value in return.

In fact, simple common sense also makes it obvious that a stronger man is less likely to be injured in any given situation...and that a more flexible man is also less prone to injury.

Many years ago, when I first started flying, a student pilot was required to practice spins and proper recovery from spins. Then somebody decided that more people were killed as a result of such training than as a result of accidental spins. Whereupon, they stopped teaching students spins and spin recovery.

Now, somebody has suddenly noticed that quite a large number of supposedly well-trained pilots are killing themselves as a result of accidental spins...probably because they do not know what to do if an accidental spin occurs; never having been taught the proper procedure.

In such situations, it is almost impossible to come up with anything even approaching a reliable set of statistics...and I will personally be very surprised if any meaningful statistics are ever produced to indicate the actual value of exercise for the purpose of preventing injuries. Therefore, in such cases, we must simply rely on common sense, self-evident truth, obvious fact...call it what you may.

An injury occurs when a *force* is imposed upon a muscle (or a joint) to the degree that the *force* exceeds the *breaking strength* of the body part, the muscle or joint. That much is undeniable...and thus, it follows that the injury would *not* have occurred if the breaking strength had been greater than the force.

If a rope has a breaking strength of 100 pounds, then it will not break as a result of 50 pounds of force. But if its breaking strength is only 40 pounds, then 50 pounds of force must break it.

A coach can do little or nothing to reduce the forces that will be imposed upon his athletes on the field. But, he certainly can increase the breaking strength of their muscles and joints.

In some cases, the forces will be so great that no possible level of human strength would be high enough to prevent injury...but even in these cases, the extent of the injury may well be reduced as a result of exercise-developed strength. Thus, exercise will reduce the level of damage in many cases...as well as prevent injury in many cases.

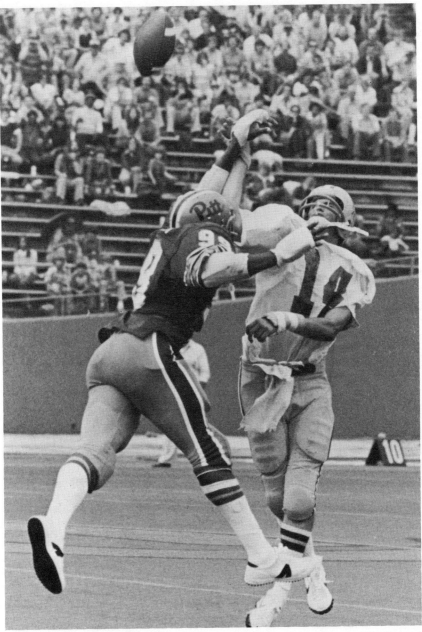

A coach can do little or nothing to reduce the forces that will be imposed upon his athlete on the field. But he certainly can increase the breaking strength of their muscles and joints.

Avoiding and Preventing Injuries

So much for *preventing* injury...even in the lack of statistics to prove the value of exercise for the purpose of preventing injury, it is obvious that exercise does help prevent injury, and it also reduces the extent of damage in many other cases.

But we still need to look at the subject of *avoiding injury*. We need to be aware of the factors that cause most training injuries, the type of injuries that are directly caused by exercise. Almost all of these injuries could easily be avoided.

Again...such injuries result when the force exceeds the breaking strength of a muscle or a joint. Therefore, the force that is involved in exercise should be as low as possible without reducing the productivity of the exercise.

At first glance, this may appear to present a paradox...since exercise consists of exposing muscles and joints to force. But in fact, no paradox exists...it is easily possible to produce the maximum possible strength from exercise while avoiding at least a large part of the force that is usually involved in exercise. Unrequired force does absolutely nothing in the way of increasing strength, while causing almost all injuries that are a direct result of exercise.

Bad form, or style of performance is the culprit in almost all such cases...and this usually involves sudden, jerky movement. Jerking greatly increases the forces imposed on the muscles and joints.

But in practice, thousands of athletes train in what may well be the most dangerous manner...meanwhile believing that their style of training is quite safe. *And*...meanwhile they avoid the most productive part of their exercises under the totally mistaken impression that they are thereby helping to avoid injury. So they train in a dangerous manner, while considering it safe...and avoid a productive style of training because they wrongly consider it dangerous.

Most people are absolutely convinced that a *hard* exercise is a *dangerous* exercise...and sometimes, in a few special situations, this may be true. But in most situations encountered in exercise, it is exactly the opposite of the truth...it is utterly false.

Remember...force causes injuries.

It matters not at all how hard it *feels*...all that matters is the force in relation to the breaking strength. Since we are never aware of the exact, momentary breaking strength...all we can do is reduce the force as much as possible while still working the muscles as hard as possible.

And again there is no paradox involved, as the following example will clearly prove.

If an athlete walks into the gymnasium with the momentary ability to curl 150 pounds...and if he actually curls 150 pounds...then he will be working as hard as he can at that point in time...and he will also be producing maximum possible force.

And if it happens that the momentary breaking strength of his tendons is only 140 pounds...then he will injure himself. Under these circumstances, injury is unavoidable.

But instead, if the athlete used a barbell weighing only 120 pounds...and if he performed several repetitions with this lighter weight...and if the form was good and the movement fairly slow...then he would probably never produce more than 125 pounds of force, which would be *less* than the breaking strength of his tendons...and the injury that was unavoidable with 150 pounds is thus avoided.

During the first repetition with this lighter weight, the resistance would *feel* light...because, at this point in the exercise, the resistance would be well below the momentary strength level of the athlete's muscles.

During later repetitions, the same resistance would feel much heavier, much *harder*...but in fact, the weight has not changed. All that has changed is the athlete's momentary strength, which has been reduced as a result of the first few, seemingly light, repetitions.

And when he reaches the final repetition, it will feel very heavy indeed...but again, the weight remains the same.

In fact, if the exercise is performed from first to last in good form, then the actual force will be lowest in the final repetition because the speed of movement will be less at that point.

Therefore, the final, seemingly hardest, repetition will feel very *hard*...and it is probably only natural for people to feel that it is the most dangerous rep-

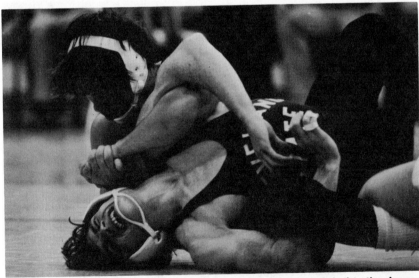

An injury occurs when a force is imposed on a muscle (or a joint) to the degree that the force exceeds the breaking strength of the body part, the muscle or joint. That much is undeniable...and thus it follows that the injury would not have occurred if the breaking strength had been greater than the force.

etition, because it feels that way. But in fact, it is the safest repetition in the exercise...because, at that point in the exercise the athlete is no longer strong enough to produce a force high enough to hurt himself, at least if he avoids jerking.

As a result of the widespread misunderstanding that exists in regard to these very simple points...misunderstanding that has probably resulted from the fact that nobody ever bothered to consider the involved factors in the light of physical law...most athletes avoid the final, seemingly hardest repetitions. Mistakenly they believe they are thus avoiding injury; when, in fact, all they are avoiding is the most important and most productive part of the exercises, and the safest part as well.

Exercise builds strength by exposing muscles to an *overload*...to a level of work that is beyond the limits of momentary ability, or, at least, well inside the existing level of reserve ability...far beyond the limits of normal activity.

But it is neither necessary nor desirable to expose a muscle to a maximum work load when it is fresh and strong...and doing so is dangerous.

If, instead, the muscle is *pre-exhausted* by the performance of several repetitions against a resistance that is well below the starting level of strength...then, later in the exercise, when a point of muscular failure is reached, the forces involved will be greatly reduced.

Upon reaching a point of momentary muscular failure, the resistance will certainly feel much heavier than it did at the start of the exercise...but that is merely an illusion produced by the fact that the athlete's *momentary* ability has declined to the point that he is unable to produce enough force to move the weight.

In the example given, involving a curl with 120 pounds, 125 pounds of force might have been produced during each of the first few repetitions...but at the end of the set, when movement is momentarily impossible, the athlete may be producing only 110 pounds of force, or less.

And, if 125 pounds of force did not hurt him...then 110 pounds of force certainly will not hurt him, regardless of how it *feels* at the moment.

The breaking strength of a muscle (or tendon, or joint) does not decline during an exercise...it remains unchanged. All that happens is that an athlete's muscles become progressively weaker until they reach a point where it is impossible for them to continue with the available resistance.

If an injury is going to be produced by an exercise, then it will usually occur during the first few repetitions...simply because the forces are higher at that point in the exercise.

With the exception of weight lifters, athletes should *never* be required to lift as much weight as possible for a single maximum attempt repetition...such lifts are not required for building maximum strength, and they greatly increase the danger of injury.

7
Preventing Injuries in Sports

By Arthur Jones

Injuries are produced by force...a force that exceeds the structural integrity of the body. When a force is encountered that exceeds the *breaking strength* of the body, then an injury literally must be produced. Only two factors are involved...1) the force that *produces* the injury...and 2) the strength of the body that *permits* injury. Obviously, injuries can be avoided by either of two methods; by lowering the force...or by increasing the strength of the body.

Protective equipment (pads, helmets, etc.) are provided for athletes involved in sports that involve contact...the only purpose of such equipment is an attempt to reduce the forces imposed upon the body. So reducing the force is an approach to safety that is already in use.

But very little in the way of worthwhile efforts is being made in the direction of solving the problem of safety in the only other way possible; not much is being done to increase the structural strength of the body.

Properly conducted exercise is capable of greatly increasing the structural integrity of an atnlete...the result being an athlete who will be far less likely to suffer an injury.

Proper exercise will increase the strength of the muscles, connective tissues (ligaments and tendons), and even the bones...and will also increase the possible range of movement or flexibility. All of these results will greatly reduce the chances of injury.

Up to this point in time, most of the attention given to exercise has been for the purpose of increasing functional ability...hoping for increases in strength or speed, or both, and exercise is certainly capable of producing such results; very worthwhile results that will improve the performance of any

77

athlete in any sport...but exercise can (and should) produce these increases in functional ability while simultaneously reducing the chances of injury.

Exercise can help prevent injuries...and exercise *should* help prevent injuries; but in practice, it sometimes causes injuries...causes injuries in one or both of two ways. Training injuries are usually obvious. The cause and effect are so closely related that the fault is apparent...if, for example, a muscle is pulled while performing an exercise, then the blame is easy to place; but *indirect* injuries are not so easy to see, and may easily be blamed on something else.

If, for example, a hamstring is pulled during a football game, then it may not occur to the coach that the real fault exists in the weight room and not on the field. Hamstring pulls can, and frequently do, result from an improper program of exercise. If the muscles of the frontal thigh are greatly strengthened while little or no attention is given to training the rear of the thigh, then you are literally asking for trouble. Or, if the strength of the hamstrings is increased while nothing is done for the flexibility, then again you are asking for trouble.

In the first instance (no exercise for the hamstrings), the muscles of the frontal thigh may become so strong that they are capable of producing a

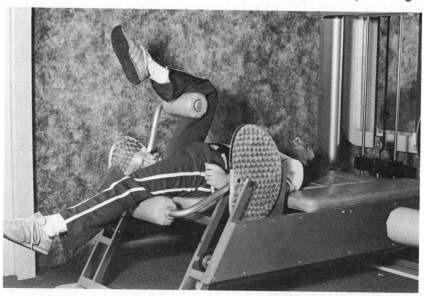

Proper exercise will increase the strength of the muscles, connective tissues (ligaments and tendons), and even the bones...and will also increase the possible range of movement, or flexibilty. All of these results will greatly reduce the chances of injury.

force which exceeds the structural integrity of the hamstrings...in which case, the hamstrings may be torn loose from their connective tissue, or a rupture of the muscle itself may result.

In the second case (strength but no flexibility in the hamstrings), an encountered force may pull the hamstring beyond its possible range of movement...with the same result, damage to the connective tissue or the muscle itself, or both.

Such injuries (and a long list of other possible injuries) should properly be blamed on a poor exercise program...but they seldom are, because most of these injuries do not occur in the weight room; do not occur until later...at which point the cause and effect situation is no longer obvious.

An exercise program should be *balanced*...the strength of the muscles on both sides of all joints should be increased in proportion. And full range exercises should be used in order to insure great flexibility.

So-called *explosive movements* should be avoided like the plague for several reasons...primarily because such a style of training is very poor for the purpose of building strength...and, secondarily, because it is extremely dangerous.

On the football field or the basketball court, a player must move suddenly...but in the weight room such sudden movement is the worst thing one can do. Weights should be *lifted*...not *thrown.* When a weight is moved suddenly it is *not being lifted*...instead, it is being thrown. The involved muscles give the weight a sudden jerk at the start of the movement...and then, during the balance of the movement, the muscles are not in the slightest way involved.

The result is that a small part of the muscle is exposed to a very dangerous jerk...and the largest part of the muscle is exposed to nothing except the danger of injury.

Building strength is one thing...*demonstrating strength* is an entirely different matter, particularly if the lifting of weight is used as a demonstration of strength.

A few individuals have recently gone to great lengths in efforts to promote so-called explosive training. Such training will afford little or nothing of value, and will probably produce a number of injuries that should have been avoided.

How fast one moves while performing exercises for the purpose of building strength has *absolutely nothing* to do with how fast one can move while using the strength of those same muscles. So training slowly certainly will *not* make one *slow.* And training fast certainly will *not* make one *fast*...on the contrary, fast training may well stop one from moving at all.

By *fast* training we simply mean the actual speed of movement...not the length of the workout. Workouts should be quite brief (or fast), but during the

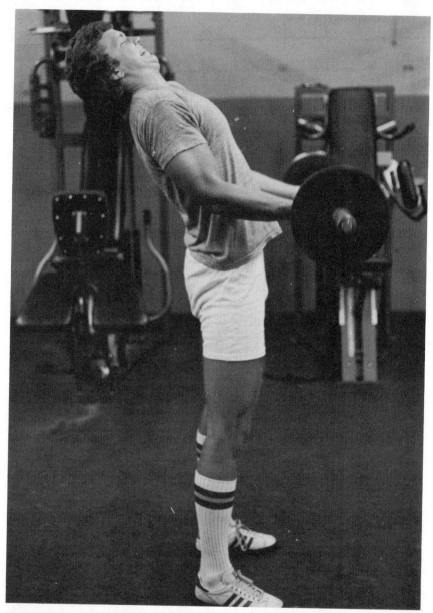

Weights should be lifted...not thrown. When a weight is moved suddenly it is not being lifted...instead, it is being thrown. The involved muscles give the weight a sudden jerk at the start of the movement...and then, during the balance of the movement, the muscles are not in the slightest way involved.

workout all movements should be performed fairly slowly...sudden movement and jerking should be avoided entirely.

We have conducted much research, and at the moment, we are planning several more large-scale research projects in conjunction with major universities...the results of which will be published—win, lose or draw.

In the meantime, do not be misled...regardless of what type of equipment is used, barbells, universal-type machines or Nautilus machines, do all that is possible to assure that the athletes perform their exercises in very strict style, with fairly slow movement and with a definite pause at both ends of all movements.

At the moment, a motion picture is being produced that clearly shows *exactly* what happens when an exercise is performed in a fast manner...at a filming speed of 14,000 frames per second it becomes possible to see what is really happening, as opposed to what one may *think* is happening. The difference is literally shocking. The same film will also show what happens during an exercise movement performed at a *proper speed*, which is a fairly slow speed. For the first time it will be possible actually to see and compare the differences.

Exercise can go a long way in the direction of preventing injury...and it should...and it will, when the simple truth is widely known.

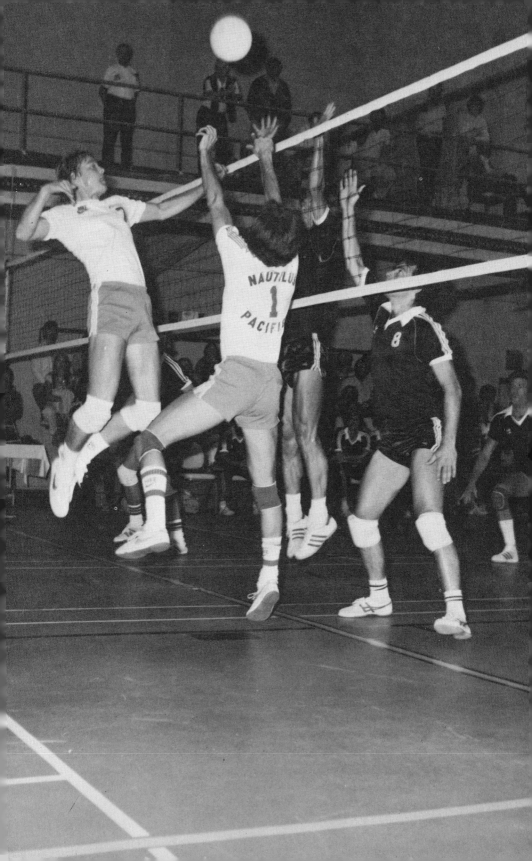

8
Improving Functional Ability In Any Sport

By Arthur Jones

Human performance is a product of five factors...1) bodily proportions, 2) neurological efficiency, 3) cardiovascular ability, 4) skill, and 5) muscular strength. All of these factors are important, but it should be clearly understood that only one factor is actually productive; the other four being supportive in nature.

Ideal bodily proportions for a particular activity may be almost entirely responsible for a championship performance...if the other four factors are at least average; but, bodily proportions perform no work on their own; their contribution to performance consists of providing the working muscles with an advantage in leverage.

Superior neurological efficiency is also important for a high level of performance...but again, it performs no work itself; it merely permits work with a higher than average degree of efficiency.

Cardiovascular ability is an absolute requirement for life itself...and a lack of this ability will certainly prevent a high level of performance; yet...no amount of cardiovascular ability will perform work. Movement is produced only by the working muscles.

Skill may well be the single most imnportant factor in any activity; but skill cannot perform work. What it does do is provide the working muscles with the ability to work at a higher level of efficiency...it channels the force produced by the muscles into a proper direction, and helps to prevent the waste of energy involved in an unskilled performance.

All of the first four factors are important, but none of them do the slightest amount of work. The fifth factor is the only one that is actually productive...all of the others help, but only the muscles perform work.

When the previously mentioned points are understood, it becomes obvious that the five factors should be divided into two categories...four *supportive* factors in one category...and one *productive* factor in the other category.

And...the same five factors should also be divided into two other categories, since two of the five factors are determined by genetics and three factors can be improved. So our attention and efforts should be restricted to the three factors that can be improved.

Absolutely nothing can be done to improve either bodily proportions or neurological efficiency. We must do the best we can with what we have...these factors are either good or bad, but are outside our realm of control in any case.

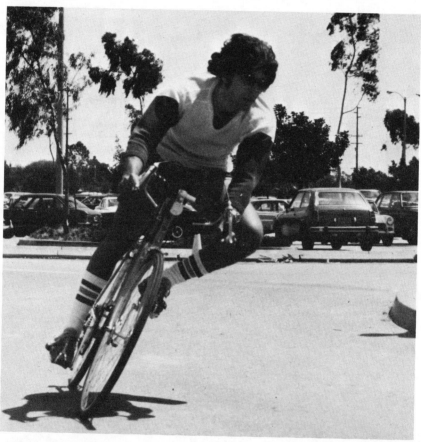

How fast one moves while performing exercises for the purpose of building strength has absolutely nothing to do with how fast one can move while using the strength of those same muscles.

But we can do something about the other three factors...these can be improved, and should be. At this point in the history of sports, a very high percentage of training is devoted to the improvement of skill...and it should be, since skill is probably the single most important factor in most activities. Cardiovascular ability is also given a great deal of attention...and again, it should be, since a lack of at least adequate cardiovascular ability will certainly limit performance.

In a sense, cardiovascular ability is linked very closely to skill...since skill results only from the practice of a particular activity. This activity will also help to produce the required level of cardiovascular ability. Skill in basketball, for example, is produced only by playing basketball...and the level of cardiovascular ability required for basketball is produced by the same training.

Additionally, most athletes also practice some form of training that is intended only for the purpose of increasing cardiovascular activity...so in most sports cardiovascular ability is given the degree of attention that it deserves.

Thus, in practice, two of our three improvable factors are already receiving the attention they require...while one improvable factor remains largely neglected. And, the neglected factor just happens to be the only productive factor on the list...the only factor capable of producing movement, the only factor able to perform work. Muscular strength is the neglected factor.

Muscular strength, I am tempted to say, is almost the *feared factor*...and it is certainly the *misunderstood factor*...a misunderstanding based entirely on superstition, ignorance, and outright fraud.

The power-train in an automobile consists of several related parts...all of which are important, but only one of which is actually productive. The engine produces power, and power is transmitted by the transmission...to the drive shaft...to the differential...and, finally, to the axle. The power produced by the engine cannot be used without the help of the other required parts of the power-train; but only the engine actually produces power...only the engine performs work...only the engine provides energy...only the engine produces movement.

The power-train in a human works much the same...several factors are required for performance; but only one factor is actually productive...only the muscles produce power...only the muscles perform work...only the muscles produce movement.

When considering an automobile, most people are clearly aware of the importance of a powerful engine...yet many of the same people fail to realize that powerful muscles are equally important in a man. In fact, the situation is actually worse than that...many people, probably most people, are literally afraid of powerful muscles; afraid in the sense that they sincerely believe powerful muscles will somehow limit their performance, reduce their functional ability. Such fear is based on superstition, with no basis of fact; but it is a common fear, a widespread fear, a well-established fear, a sincerely believed fear...and being so well established, it is a fear that is difficult to remove with the light of reason.

So we will be stuck with the results of such a groundless fear for a long time into the future, perhaps forever...thousands of injuries will be produced that could have been prevented, much pain will be suffered that could easily have been prevented, and the level of human performance will remain lower than it could have been and should have been.

Thus we have already paid, are now paying, and will continue to pay a very high price as a result of fear based entirely on ignorance.

Individuals vary, on a gross scale...but a particular individual will reach his own limit of functional ability only when all three of the improvable factors are improved as much as possible. Additional improvement is possible only when skill, cardiovascular ability, and strength have all been raised to the highest possible level consistent with the requirements of a particular sport.

Yet, in the real world, we have a situation where literally thousands of coaches and millions of athletes are doing little or nothing in the way of improving strength...usually because they are actually afraid to increase strength; afraid they will reduce the speed of movement, or flexibility...afraid they will somehow limit functional ability. All of these fears are utterly without foundation...all of these fears are based on false beliefs that are the exact opposite of the truth.

Stronger muscles will make an athlete *faster*, not slower, in any sport...proper strength training will actually increase his flexibiity, in any area of movement...greater strength will improve his functional ability in any activity related to sports.

And greater muscular strength will go a long way in the direction of preventing injuries.

So, in sports, exercise remains the neglected factor...a neglect largely resulting from fear, a fear based on ignorance. Sometimes in the far distant future, people will probably look back on the present era of sports as the age of ignorance...primarily because of the lack of attention now being given to the intelligent use of exercise. Most athletes still finish their careers with absolutely nothing in the way of strength training...and very few (if any) athletes are producing even 50 percent of the potential benefit of a properly conducted program of exercise.

Well under two hours of total time devoted to proper exercise on a weekly basis will produce 100 percent of the potential benefits of strength training...three weekly workouts of less than 40 minutes each are all that are required; longer workouts, or more frequent workouts, are neither necessary nor desirable.

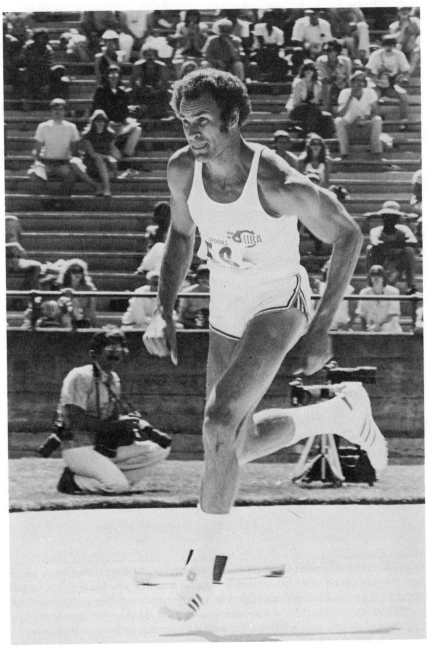

Stronger muscles will make an athlete faster, not slower, in any sport...

Exercise performed for the purpose of increasing strength should be brief, infrequent, and of very high intensity...as *hard* as momentarily possible; carried to a point of momentary muscular failure. Conducted in this fashion, strength training not only can be brief but literally must be brief; more than three such weekly workouts would actually result in a reduction of strength instead of an increase.

But again, superstition rears its ugly head...common belief tends to equate *more* with better...in effect, if *some* is good then *more* must be even better; which may be true in some things; but which certainly is not true in the case of proper strength training. The widespread result of this myth is that the few people who do train for strength almost always train far too much...and seldom train with a high enough level of intensity.

So even the few people who are aware of the potential benefit of proper exercise, usually miss the mark by a wide margin...another result of ignorance; in this instance the ignorance being a result of a lack of accurate knowledge, rather than a belief in a baseless fear.

As a result of the widespread fear of exercise and a lack of factual information on the subject of exercise, most coaches and athletes are overlooking a very important factor...while continuing to labor under the mistaken belief that they are doing *everything possible* in the direction of improving functional ability. The *edge* that most coaches are constantly looking for has been in plain sight for a long time...but remains largely untapped, unsuspected, even feared, and certainly misunderstood.

Nothing previously mentioned should be misunderstood to imply that strength is the most important factor...and there is no implication that the other factors are unimportant. On the contrary, the importance of proper bodily proportions for a particular activity is so great that this one factor may be the difference between a champion and an utter failure...with little or no regard for the other factors.

Likewise, skill is almost always the most important factor in any activity. And neurological efficiency, or a lack of it, can easily be the difference between success and failure. And, of course, at least adequate cardiovascular ability is required for any activity.

...Common belief tends to equate more with better...in effect, if some is good then more must be even better which may be true in some things; but which certainly is not true in the case of proper strength training. The widespread result of this myth is that the few people who do train for strength almost always train far too much...and seldom train with a high enough level of intensity.

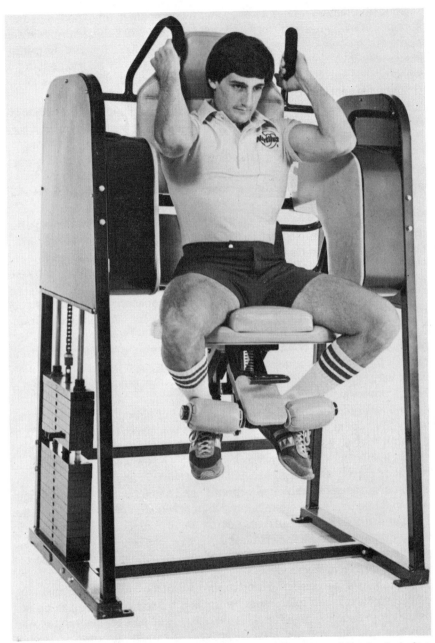

But, regardless of the sport, and regardless of the area of the body being trained...certain basic rules must be applied if good results are to be expected from exercise performed for the purpose of increasing strength.

So all the factors are important...and a champion in any sport is usually superior in every respect; with perhaps one exception...his strength is seldom what it could be, almost never as high as it should be, and his performance will thus be less than his real potential. He may be the best in the world...but if his strength is not as high as possible, then he has never reached the real limit of his individual ability.

Until this simple truth is clearly understood and accepted...until the obvious implications are applied in practice...functional ability will remain less than it could have been.

Strength is *general*...the application of strength is selective; the proper use of strength in any activity comes only from the practice of the particular activity. Skill is required for the proper use of strength, and skill is produced in only one way...through the practice of a particular activity.

Gymnastics may well produce the strength required for swimming...but the skill required to use that strength for swimming can come only from swimming itself. And no amount of skill at swimming will move a swimmer through the water without the strength to move his limbs...and his limbs are moved by the strength of his muscles.

The proper development of skill requires the application of a great deal of time to the practice of a particular activity...and such a large amount of training literally prevents the utilization of high intensity training methods. The result is that training conducted for the development of skill is not the best type of training for increasing strength. Proper strength training must involve very high intensity...which literally can neither be practiced frequently nor for prolonged periods.

So a swimmer will build a certain amount of strength from swimming, while developing skill at swimming...but he will never build the degree of strength that is actually helpful to a champion swimmer; will never build such a level of strength from swimming itself. And the same thing applies to a football player, a basketball player or an athlete in any sport.

Some sports demand *overall* strength...and some sports require strength only in some areas; for example, a gymnast requires great strength in the torso and arm muscles...but does not require an equal degree of strength in the legs; whereas, a football player needs overall strength.

So exercise should be applied selectively, depending upon the sport in which an athlete is involved.

But, regardless of the sport, and regardless of the area of the body being trained; certain basic rules must be applied if good results are to be expected from exercise performed for the purpose of increasing strength. And here we get into another area of widespread myth...an area of misunderstanding that literally prevents the production of good results from exercise in many cases.

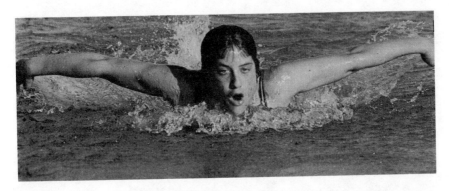

A swimmer can build a certrain amount of strength from swimming, while developing skill at swimming...but she will never build the degree of strength that is actually helpful to a champion swimmer; will never build such a level of strength from swimming itself. And the same thing applies to a football player, a basketball player or an athlete in any sport.

Without attempting to become involved in a lengthy refutation of any of the many common misconceptions in this area, the rules for proper exercise can be stated very briefly; use full-range exercises to assure development of the entire length of the involved muscles, and to increase flexibility...perform all movements in a rather slow fashion, avoid all sudden movements or jerking, and pause briefly at both ends of all movements...continue the exercise to a point of momentary muscular failure, this point should be reached after 10 to 12 repetitions working against as much resistance as possible...pay careful attention to the form, or style of performance, and do not permit the form to deteriorate in an effort to use more resistance or increase the number of possible repetitions...increase the resistance whenever possible, but not until more resistance can be handled with a sacrifice in form.

Properly performed, only one *set* of each of 10 to 12 exercises will produce very good results in almost all cases...multiple sets are seldom if ever required for the purpose of increasing strength, as long as each exercise is continued to a point of momentary failure in good form.

If several sets of an exercise are used, then it quickly becomes literally impossible for an athlete to involve maximum intensity in each set...and attempting to do so will produce losses in strength instead of gains; so multiple sets are neither necessary nor desirable in most cases...the primary exception is a competitive weight lifter who obviously must develop skill as well as strength, the skill required to lift a weight in a particular fashion.

An athlete should not be misled by advice to the effect that he must train *explosive strength*...such a style of training is the least productive style of training possible, and by far the most dangerous style of training.

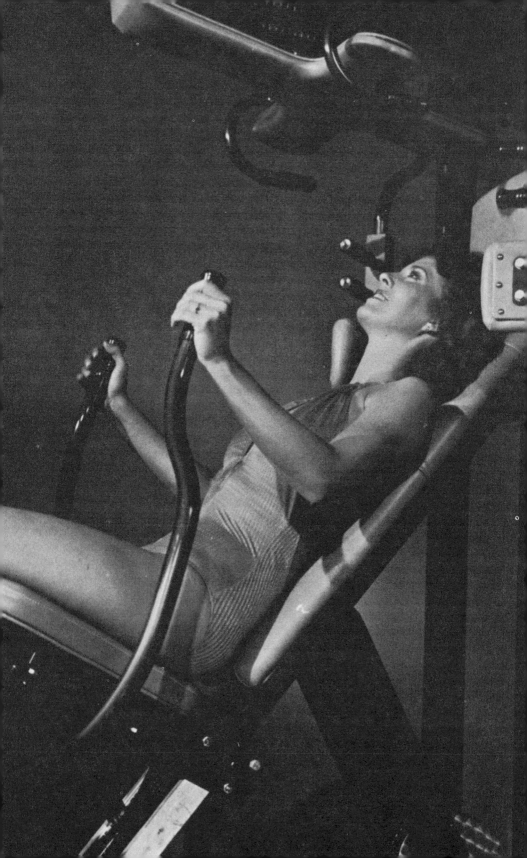

9
Negative Work As a Factor In Exercise

By Arthur Jones

When an exerciser lifts a weight, his muscles are performing positive work...or in a language of physiologists, concentric contraction is occurring. Muscles are producing movement by reducing their length. A common example of positive work is provided by the lifting portion of a bench press.

Negative work, or eccentric contraction, is produced when an exerciser lowers a weight...when the downward movement of a weight is limited by the action of muscles.

In either case, the exerciser's muscles are working...during positive work, the muscles are working to lift a weight against the force of gravity...and during negative work the muscles are still working against the force of gravity by preventing the normal acceleration that would result if the weight was simply dropped.

Most forms of exercise involve both positive and negative work...only recently has it become possible to perform a style of exercise that involves only positive work, a type of exercise that totally removes the negative part of the work. Since the introduction of such positive-only forms of exercise, a great deal of controversy has arisen concerning the relative merits of positive and negative work. The primary result is great confusion on the part of many coaches and athletes.

Nearly 40 years ago when I visited the Texas Centennial in 1936, I first became aware of one of the results of negative work...a result that surprised me at the time, and a result that I then did not understand. My brother and I rode the elevator to the top floor of the tallest building in Dallas (30-odd stories) and walked back down to street level...the following day I was so sore I could barely walk.

Negative Work As a Factor In Exercise

Walking down stairs involves almost pure negative work, and it was the negative work that made me sore...if instead I had climbed the stairs and then returned to street level on the elevator, I would have experienced little or nothing in the way of muscular soreness; because, in this case, the work would have been almost pure positive work...and the positive part of work produces very little or no muscular soreness.

Why? In what way is negative work different from positive work to the extent that one produces considerable muscular soreness while the other produces almost no soreness?

I cannot answer that question. But I am clearly aware that such a difference exists. And there are other differences...some of which are obvious...but most of which are not so obvious. But most of these other differences are easily understood once they have been pointed out in simple language, which is the purpose of this article.

One obvious difference is the effect upon cardiopulmonary activity; climbing stairs, performing positive work, will quickly elevate both the rate of breathing and the heart rate...while going down stairs, performing negative work, will have a much lower effect in these areas. So it is immediately apparent that negative work is not of much value for the purpose of increasing cardiovascular (or cardiopulmonary) condition.

So far it might appear that negative work is thus left with the short end of the stick...since it causes a great deal of muscular soreness and is of little value for cardiovascular conditioning purposes; but a clear look at the whole picture gives an opposite impression...and when all of the facts are considered, it then becomes obvious that negative work is certainly the most important part of exercises performed for a wide variety of purposes.

For example...pre-stretching, the neurological stimulation required for a high intensity of muscular contraction, is a result of negative work; so a truly high intensity of muscular work is impossible without negative work...and exercises performed for the purpose of building strength are of very little value without a high intensity of work.

Third...full range exercise designed to work the entire length of a muscular structure also requires negative work; to provide the back pressure of force that is required in a finishing position of full muscular contraction.

Fourth...negative work makes it possible to exercise a muscle that is too weak to move against the slightest resistance. Thus negative work is a very valuable tool for the purpose of working muscles that have become weak as a result of injury.

So the facts are plain; there is a place for both positive and negative work...the relative value of one or the other type is being determined by the purpose for which exercises are being performed. If flexibility, strength or full-range exercise is an exerciser's goal, then he must provide negative

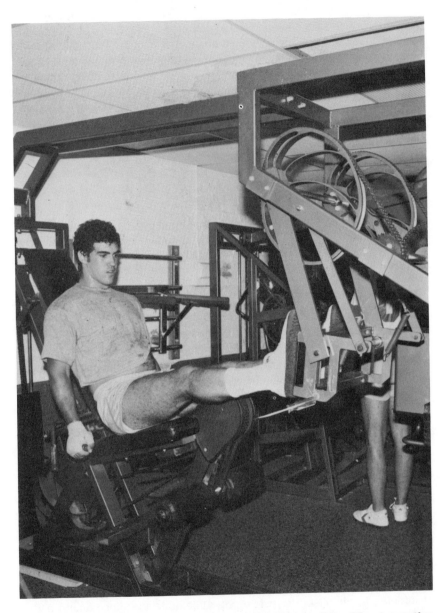

A truly high intensity level of muscular work is impossible without negative work...and exercises performed for the purpose of building strength are of very little value without a high intensity of work.

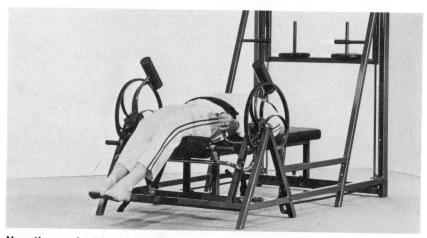

Negative work makes it possible to exercise a muscle that is too weak to move against even the slightest resistance. Thus negative work is a very valuable tool for the purpose of working muscles that have become weak as a result of injury.

work as a part of his exercise...if he is interested only in cardiovascular conditioning, then negative work is not required.

Approximately three years ago we conducted a large number of lengthy tests that involved pure negative work...negative-only exercise; the positive part of the work was entirely removed. We wanted to see just what would happen to subjects exposed to such a form of exercise. But it should be clearly understood that these tests were not conducted because we felt that positive work was somehow bad...rather, it was necessary to eliminate the positive work only in order to be sure that the results produced were in fact a product of negative work. If both positive and negative work were mixed, it would then have been impossible to say which result was produced by which type of work.

I also want to point out that such a style of training is certainly not a practical style of exercise because it requires a large number of willing helpers; assistants are needed to lift the weight so that the test subject can perform only the negative part of the work by lowering a weight that was first lifted by his helpers.

As test subjects, we used several professional football players, a number of athletes in other sports, a few non-athletes, and, after gaining a few months of experience with these trainees, I tried a negative-only workout program myself. The results in every single case can only be described as outstanding; growth was rapid in all subjects, and strength increases came much more rapidly than we expected.

Negative Work As a Factor In Exercise

Only three workouts were conducted each week, and in several cases we used approximately 10 exercises during each workout, some subjects performed only 8 or 9 exercises during each training period and a few subjects performed as many as a dozen different exercises.

Seven to 10 repetitions were performed during each *set* of an exercise...and we increased the resistance when it was possible to perform as many as 10 repetitions in good form.

Only one *set* of each exercise was performed; thus, an entire workout might consist of as few as 56 repetitions...7 repetitions of each of 8 exercises. And a maximum length workout would be not more than 120 repetitions...10 repetitions of each of 12 exercises.

Performed in the style that we did them during these test programs, a set of an exercise requires approximately two minutes...and we used very little or no rest between exercises...thus an entire workout usually required approximately 18 to 20 minutes, and never much if any more than 30 minutes. Barbells, exercise machines and Nautilus machines were used as equipment during these test programs...and we restricted our attention to basic exercises involving large muscular structures; pullover exercises performed in a Nautilus machine, hip and back exercises in a Nautilus machine, biceps and triceps exercises both performed in a Nautilus machine, chinning and dipping exercises performed on a conventional machine, and seated presses, bench presses, and shoulder shrugs all performed with a barbell. A few other exercises were performed at times by some subjects, but the exercises listed were the prime movements involved.

In addition to the weight exercises listed, the athletes also ran for 12 minutes on the same day that they trained with weights, running immediately after the weight workout. Thus their entire training required a total of approximately two hours.

As mentioned previously, such programs prove to be impractical for the use of a large number of subjects simply and only because a large number of helpers were required to lift the weights, and it became increasingly difficult to recruit willing helpers in great enough numbers. Secondly, some of our subjects became so strong that it was literally impossible to lift as much weight as they could properly lower; with the tools we had at our disposal, it was not possible to get enough people into a proper position to lift a really heavy weight...for example, one subject reached a point where he was using 1,400 pounds on a Nautilus Hip and Back machine, and we could not get helpers around the machine to lift that amount of weight.

That particular problem was eventually solved by using a 500-pound weight stack on the machine, and by adding the weight of a 200-pound man standing on the weight stack after it had been lifted by the helpers...and then by having the test subject use the machine one leg at a time.

Negative Work As a Factor In Exercise

Another problem was caused by the fact that helpers would not always release the weight simultaneously...the result being that the weight would be released unevenly, causing too much weight to be placed on one arm (or leg) while no weight was on the other limb. So great caution must be used during the hand-off of the weight; if not, the subject might drop the weight and an injury could result. We had no injuries with any of our subjects, but we quickly learned to be very careful with the hand-off of the weights.

Since it is possible to use far more than a normal amount of weight when performing negative-only exercises, this also presented a problem...it was impossible, for example, to load enough weight onto a barbell for some of the exercises. And, during the shoulder shrugs, it was impossible for the test subjects to retain a grip on the bar with their hands if the weight was as heavy as really required; in that case, the problem was solved by strapping the hands to the bar.

In all cases, we used as much weight as possible...determining the correct amount of weight by simple trial and error; selecting an amount of weight that the subjects could handle properly for at least 7 (but not more than 10) repetitions.

Speed of movement was quite slow; the subjects permitted the weight to move slowly to the bottom position, resisting this movement and not permitting the weight to drop suddenly...a normal repetition required approximately 10 to 15 seconds for the lowering portion of the exercises. During the first 2 or 3 repetitions, it would have been possible for the subjects to stop the downward movement of the weight...but no attempt to stop the movement was made; instead, the weight was permitted to move constantly, but very slowly.

After a few repetitions, if the weight was selected correctly, it was then impossible to stop the downward movement...and from that point until the end of the exercise, the subject tried as hard as possible to stop the movement. An exercise was finished only when the subject was trying as hard as possible to stop the downward movement, but couldn't...and the entire movement was completed in about 2 or 3 seconds in spite of the subject's best efforts to stop the movement.

So a properly performed set of an exercise consisted of a few repetitions during which the subject could have stopped the movement, but did not try...followed by a few more repetitions during which he was trying as hard as possible to stop the movement, but failing.

The weight should be impossible to lift, but possible to *hold* motionless in any position during the movement.

Altogether, we performed several *man years* of such training over a period of approximately six months; the results were outstanding in all cases, and we learned a great deal about the actual value of the negative

98

part of exercise. Since these first experiments, we have continued to test various combinations of training methods and styles. In the meantime, we have solved most of the original problems that we encountered during these first tests of negative-only training.

Probably the most important thing we learned is the fact that people (ourselves included) have been neglecting the negative part of exercise for years, and that their results have suffered as a consequence. So pay careful attention to both the positive and the negative parts of exercises; lift the weight steadily, smoothly, and fairly slowly...and then lower the weight back down to the starting position even more slowly. Doing exercises in this fashion will cause an exerciser to reduce the number of repetitions or the amount of weight, or both...but it will greatly increase his results, and that is what he is after. And, as a side benefit, such a style of training will almost totally eliminate the chance of injury.

...and when all of the facts are considered, it then becomes obvious that negative work is certainly the most important part of exercises performed for a wide variety of purposes.

10
Negative Accentuated Strength Training

By Arthur Jones

In the previous chapter, I covered briefly the subject of *negative* strength. I mentioned several of the advantages and several of the problems connected with such a style of training. Very briefly, again, the advantages provided by the negative part of exercise are...1) stretching, for the improvement of flexibility...2) pre-stretching, for a high intensity of muscular contraction...3) resistance in the position of full contraction, for full-range exercise...and 4) maximum application of resistance throughout a full range of possible movement, which results from the fact that it is impossible to throw a weight *down*.

The first three advantages of a negative style of training are, I think, rather obvious and easy to understand...without the back pressure of force pulling against a trainee at the start of an exercise movement, there would be nothing to stretch his muscles and improve flexibility...without such stretching of the muscles, there would also be no pre-stretch, which is the neurological stimulus required for a high intensity of muscular contraction...and, without a force pulling back against him at the end of an exercise movement, there would be no resistance in the position of full muscular contraction. Thus, without negative work, an exercise would be done for flexibility, high intensity work would be impossible, and full range exercise would be equally impossible.

The fourth advantage, however, may require a bit more of an explanation; although it is equally important, it may not be quite so obvious. While performing positive work during the *lifting* part of an exercise, it is easily possible (and common practice) to throw the weight rather than lift it. If the upwards movement is started with a jerk, or if the movement is too fast (and it usually is)...the result will be that the muscles a trainee is trying to work simply cannot keep pace with the movement of the weight. So he imposes a worthless and dangerous yank on the muscles at the start of the movement, and then the muscles contribute little or nothing to the following movement...and no benefit is derived for most of the mass of the muscles a trainee is trying to exercise.

If the weight being used is too heavy (and it usually is)...then it becomes impossible to lift the weight properly; so the trainee is forced to throw it instead of lifting it...the inevitable result being the least productive and most dangerous style of training, a style of training that will do very little except produce injuries. Now...make no mistake, the weight should be as heavy as possible; but not too heavy. It should be as heavy as a trainee can handle in good form; heavier than that and it will make good form impossible, and may produce injury...lighter than that, and a trainee is simply wasting time and burning up energy to no good purpose. So he should use as much weight as he possibly can in good form. And he should increase the weight as often and as much as he can, but do not ever increase the weight if a sacrifice in form is required to do so.

However, in the real world, it usually happens that a trainee will quickly start throwing the weight, instead of lifting it...usually under the totally mistaken impression that he is thus showing progress, since it then becomes possible to use more weight.

When a negative only style of training is practiced, however...then such throwing becomes impossible; a trainee can simply drop a weight, but he cannot throw it down.

In negative-only training, the weight is lifted for a trainee by somebody or something else...then the trainee slowly lowers the weight, performing only the negative (eccentric) part of the work. Jerking, yanking, heaving, throwing and too-fast movement are thus totally avoided...the idea is to lower the weight slowly, very slowly, but without ever quite stopping the downwards movement. At the start of a negative-only exercise a trainee should be able to stop the downwards movement if he tries...but he should not try. Then, after several repetitions (6 or 7), it should be impossible to stop the downwards movement no matter how hard he tries; but he should still be able to control it, able to maintain (but not stop) the slow, steady, smooth, downwards movement.

Then, after two or three more repetitions, a trainee should find it impossible to stop the downwards acceleration of the weight...the weight should be moving faster (not fast...simply faster than it was before), and this is when he should terminate the exercise.

If a trainee tries to go on after he finds it impossible to prevent downwards

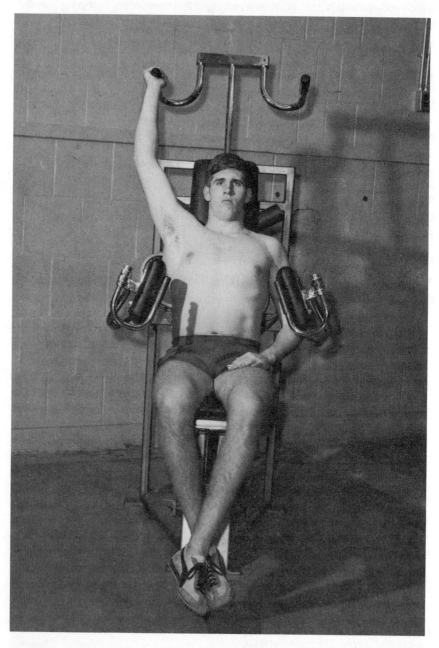

Negative accentuated training does not require helpers, and that one factor is an advantage of great importance.

acceleration of the weight, he will suddenly find himself dropping the weight...which is neither necessary nor desirable, and could be dangerous in some exercises, the bench press for example.

So, properly performed, negative-only exercise assures full range exercise for the muscles because the weight is never thrown, but always moved at a smooth, steady pace.

And that should recap the advantages of negative exercise...but there are a few problems as well; problems dealing with the practical application of negative exercise. These problems result from the fact that it is usually necessary to have somebody else lift the weight for a trainee so that he can perform only the lowering (negative) part of the exercise.

A few exercises can be performed in a negative-only fashion without help; chinning can be done by climbing into the top position with the legs so that the arms simply lower the trainee back down, and dips can be done in the same manner. Shoulder shrugs can be performed negative-only by using a bench situated just below the low point of the movement; the barbell is deadlifted from the bench while the shoulders are held in the top position of the exercise. Then after the back and legs are straight, the shoulders are slowly permitted to lower the weight. And, depending upon the availability of equipment, a few other exercises can be done in a negative-only fashion without help. But, in general, a trainee needs help; and finding such help is seldom easy; so, for most people, a totally negative program of exercises is certainly impractical.

When this problem first presented itself to us, we looked around for an answer...and the subject of this chapter, *negative accentuated* strength training, so far seems to be the best answer. Quite frankly, at this point in time, I do not know just how negative accentuated training compares to negative-only training; that is to say, I do not know which is better...or even if one actually is better. Until we have had the opportunity to conduct a large-scale comparison under good conditions and over a rather long period of time, it will remain impossible to say which is best in the sense that one style of training will produce better results than the other.

However, this is not meant to imply that I do not have an opinion at this point in time...I do; but it should be clearly understood that it is merely an opinion. I have personally trained with heavy resistance exercises of all existing kinds on a very irregular basis for a period of more than thirty-five years. This training fact really means little or nothing in itself, because such long experience can (and usually does) produce a very biased attitude; can produce a set in one's thinking, can convince him that he has nothing more to learn in regard to a particular subject. So, experience by itself means absolutely nothing; and in many cases has the result of preventing learning rather than helping it. However, it also seems to be true that little if anything of value is possible in the way of learning without experience. And it is certainly true that experience produces opinions. So, at this point in time, with no supporting evidence to base it on, my opinion is that negative accentuated training is probably as productive as negative-only training, and perhaps better in some ways.

In due course, we will conduct a careful research program in cooperation with a major university for the express purpose of comparing negative-only exercise to both negative accentuated exercise and normal exercise; but in the meantime, all I can give is an opinion...together with a few of the facts that have produced that opinion.

Negative accentuated training does *not* require helpers, and that one factor is an advantage of great importance. Second, it does not require nearly as much resistance, which is also an important consideration since a negative-only style of training sometimes requires an impossible level of resistance; more resistance than can be loaded on the bar or machine. Third, it is

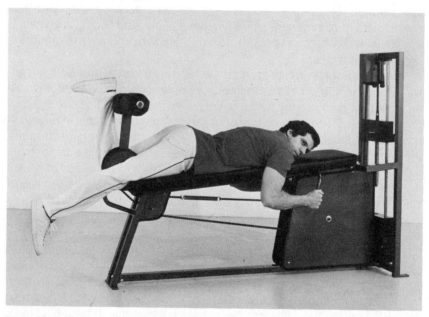

In exercise, as in most things, form (or style of performance) may not be the only thing, but it is certainly a prerequisite for good results...good form with too little weight will do little or nothing of value; but too much weight without good form is even worse, and dangerous besides.

possible to perform a much greater variety of exercises in a negative accentuated fashion.

Negative accentuated training is impossible with a barbell...not difficult, simply *impossible*. But several very good exercises can be performed on almost any type of exercise machine while using this style of training. With the conventional type machine, it is possible to perform leg presses, leg extensions, leg curls, bench presses, and standing presses...all in a negative accentuated fashion, and without help. With Nautilus machines all of the same five exercises can be performed plus curls, triceps curls, decline presses, pullovers, and hip extensions (on a Hip and Back machine).

And a trainee can do negative accentuated chins on any kind of a chinning bar, or machine that provides a chinning station. Negative accentuated dips are also possible, but not as easy to learn to do properly.

Negative accentuated exercise does *not* require more resistance than normal exercise...instead, it requires *less resistance*; but do not assume that it is thus easier; it is not...in fact, it is considerably harder than normal exercise. But the very fact that it requires less resistance is an advantage in at least two ways; in the first place, it is safer...and in the second place, it means that a trainee is far less likely to run out of available resistance, not liable to become stronger than the machine. *But again*...do not misunderstand that last statement; I did not mean to imply that a trainee will not become stronger, he certainly will become stronger, and quickly...but a negative accentuated style of training simply will not permit a trainee to use as much resistance as he can in some other ways, so the resistance available on almost any exercise machine of any kind will probably be enough to provide him with all the weight he will ever be able to handle properly in this fashion.

Using the bench press as performed on an exercise machine as an example, I will now describe the proper style of performance for negative accentuated training.

If a trainee can, for example, bench press 200 pounds for ten repetitions in a normal manner, I recommend that for negative accentuated training he use 140 pounds instead, approximately 70 percent of the weight he could lift normally.

Lift the weight in the normal fashion, but a bit more slowly than is probably done now...using both arms during the lifting (positive) part of the exercise. Then lower it slowly back down while using only one arm. Do not remove the nonworking hand from its grip, leave it in place but do not use it...permit one arm to do all the negative work by itself. Lower it *slowly*, taking approximately 8 seconds for the negative part of the exercise. Then lift it back to the top position with both arms again, using both arms equally for the lifting part of the movement. The lifting movement should be done considerably faster than the lowering part...it should only take about two seconds for the lifting part.

A trainee can easily raise it a great deal faster than that, but he should not...because he will be throwing it rather than lifting it, which is not very productive and is dangerous.

So...raise the weight with two arms, then lower it slowly with the right arm only...then raise it again with both arms, but this time lower it with the left arm, *slowly*. And so on.

Up with two, down with one, up with two again, down with the other; and this should continue until a trainee finds it impossible to raise it again. Both arms work toghether and equally during the positive part of the exercise, but work alternately during the negative part.

If the weight is selected correctly, the first three or four repetitions will seem very light...will seem far too light; but a trainee should not kid himself; by the time he reaches the eighth lifting stroke the previously light weight is correct, he should reach a point of momentary failure about the tenth repetition. After about nine lifting movements with a weight that seemed very light at the start, he should not be able to lift it up again.

When a trainee can lift it ten times in this fashion, then increase the resistance by approximately 5 percent. So a properly performed set of such an exercise should consist of approximately 8 to 10 lifting movements, plus 4 or 5 negative movements performed bt the right arm only and an equal number performed by the left arm only.

Negative accentuated chinning is performed by lifting oneself with both arms and then lowering oneself with only one arm...at first it may be necessary for him to *help himself* a bit with the nonworking arm, but rather quickly he will find that one arm can handle the negative part of a chin without help from the other arm.

Leg presses are performed by lifting the weight with both legs and then lowering it back down while using only one leg. Leg extensions and leg curls are performed in the same way.

The same rules apply to any exercise that is possible in this style, and a trainee can use this style of training with any piece of equipment that provides a stable source of resistance; he obviously cannot perform negative accentuated training with a barbell for the simple reason that he cannot release the pressure against one side of a barbell while continuing to maintain it on the other side. So do not try.

In exercise, as in most things, *form* (or style of performance) may not be the only thing, but it is certainly a prerequisite for good results...good form with too little weight will do little or nothing of value; but too much weight without good form is even worse, and dangerous besides. And a negative accentuated style of training will give a trainee both good form and outstanding results. Try it and find out.

11
Metabolic Cost of Negative Work

By Arthur Jones

A review of the literature on negative work may lead to more confusion than knowledge, primarily because anything written on the subject seems to be guilty of at least four faulty assumptions.

ONE...it has been assumed that human muscles are stronger during negative work, by comparison to their strength during positive work.

TWO...it has been assumed that the metabolic cost of negative work is much lower than the metabolic cost of positive work.

THREE...it has been assumed that negative work has very little effect upon the cardiovascular system.

FOUR...it has been assumed that the ratio of positive metabolic cost to negative metabolic cost changes as the rate of work changes.

Any or all of these four basic assumptions may be true, but they have not been proven. They have been generally accepted, I think, only because they appear to be true on the basis of rather casual observation. But even if they are true, the degree of truth involved is far less than that which has been generally accepted.

All of these four basic assumptions are based upon apparent differences and positive work. However, when several factors that have previously been ignored are considered, it is immediatey obvious that the real differences, if any, are far less than the apparent differences.

ONE, a difference in strength. While it is certainly true that an exerciser can lower more weight than he can lift, it does not necessarily follow that his muscles are actually stronger during negative work than they are during positive work.

The muscles may be stronger; but even if so, they are not as much stronger as they appear to be. The apparent gross difference in strength is, I think, primarily a result of friction...internal muscular friction.

While lifting a weight, the muscles must contract with sufficient force to move the imposed resistance...but they also have to overcome their own internal friction. Thus, during positive work, friction is working against the muscles.

Whereas, during negative work, friction is working for the muscles instead of against them.

Therefore, an exerciser's usable strength during positive work is equal to the force provided by his muscles, minus friction.,...and his usable strength during negative work is equal to the force provided by his muscles, plus friction. Friction hurts him during positive work and helps him during negative work.

It may well be that all of the difference in usable strength cannot be accounted for by friction; but even if not, it still remains true that at least part of the difference is a result of friction...thus the actual difference is certainly less than the apparent difference.

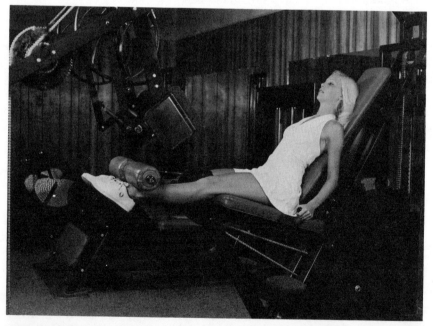

Negative work, or eccentric contraction, is produced when an exerciser lowers a weight...when the downward movement of a weight is limited by the action of muscles.

At the moment, we are conducting careful tests in an effort to determine exactly what part friction plays in the matter.

TWO, a difference in metabolic cost. A great deal of confusion exists on this point because of attempts to compare metabolic work with mechanical work, and, secondly, because of a failure to consider several related factors.

By definition, work requires movement...no movement means no work; and while this is undoubtedly true in regard to mechanical work, it certainly is not true in relation to metabolic work.

Muscles produce force, and it is easily possible for a muscle to produce a high level of force without producing movement; logically, it appears that the metabolic cost of muscular force production would be related to the level of force produced and the time that the force is maintained...rather than the amount of mechanical work performed.

If, for example, a 100-pound barbell is held motionless at the halfway position of a curling exercise, then the muscles will be required to produce a certain level of force to prevent the downward movement of the barbell. Providing that force will certainly entail metabolic cost...yet no work is involved.

Slowly, curling a 100-pound barbell also requires a greater metbolic cost than curling the same barbell at a more rapid pace; even though the amount of mechanical work involved is exactly the same in both cases.

Many other examples could be given to illustrate the same point, but it should now be obvious that attempts to relate metabolic cost to mechanical work are doomed to failure...there is no meaningful relationship. We must have another standard for comparison.

The only meaningful standard, I can think of is force/time...the amount of force produced by the muscles multiplied by the time that the force is maintained.

But again, attempts to measure force/time will be meaningless if we fail to consider friction...and will be very difficult in situations involving movement. At the moment we are working on the development of a practical means to measure accurately force/time in situations involving movement...but until and unless such equipment is produced, force/time can probably be measured accurately only in static situations.

It should be reasonably simple to determine the metabolic cost of force/time in static situations...and if this is done accurately, I think it will then be shown that a very close relationship exists between force/time and metabolic cost. Perhaps an exact relationship will be established...and if so, then we will have a standard for comparison. But in the meantime, no such standard exists; the attempt to use mechanical work as a standard for determining metabolic cost has led to widespread confusion.

When and if it becomes possible to compare the metabolic cost of negative work with that of positive work on the basis of a meaningful standard, it may well be shown that the metabolic cost is in fact exactly the same in both cases; but even if not, it will certainly be shown that the difference, if any, is far less than it is now generally assumed to be.

THREE, a difference in cardiovascular effects. When it becomes possible to determine accurately the difference, if any, between the metabolic cost of positive work and that of negative work...then, and only then, will it also be possible to make meaningful comparisons between the cardiovascular effects of positive work and those of negative work. In the meantime, any attempt to make a meaningful comparison is limited by lack of a standard for comparison.

FOUR, changing ratios of metabolic cost as a result of changes in rate of work. It is generally believed that a faster rate of work produces a high ratio of metabolic cost, and vice versa.

If, for example, two subjects are seated in the same leg press machine, in such a manner that one subject performs all of the positive work, the lifting part of the exercise, while the other subject performs all of the negative work, the lowering part of all exercise...then, at a slow rate of work, the man performing positive work might be required to pay a metabolic cost that is twice as high as the metabolic cost required of the man performing negative woprk.

But it does not follow that the actual metabolic cost is different to that degree...or even that there is any difference at all. Because the force/time factor is different...even though the speed of movement may be exactly the same with both subjects.

Remember, the man doing the positive work is lifting the resistance while also working against friction...and the man doing the negative work is lowering the resistance while being helped by friction. Thus, it could easily be possible that the man performing the positive part of the work was actually producing twice as much force/time as the other man.

But, in any case, it is obvious that the muscular work (as opposed to mechanical work) is certainly not equal... so, it is only natural that the metabolic cost would also be different.

Then, if the rate of work is increased, the apparent ratio between the metabolic cost of positive and negative work will also be changed. If, for example, the rate of work is doubled, then the apparent ratio may change from a ratio of two-to-one to a ratio of three-to-one. And again, I think that any such apparent change in ratio is an illusion resulting from a failure to consider all of the involved factors.

If, for example, the rate of work is increased by increasing the speed of movement, then a point is eventually reached where the amount of negative work involved becomes literally zero. This occurs when the downward movement of the weight is occurring at a speed equal to the normal acceleration produced by gravity, in effect, when the weight is simply dropped.

In such a situation one man would be lifting the weight fairly rapidly...while the other man would be simply dropping it, making no attempt to stop or delay the normal acceleration resulting from gravity. Obviously, then, the man doing the positive part of the work would be working...while the other man would be doing literally nothing.

Even more confusion on this point has resulted from a failure to consider basic metabolic requirements. A man at rest is constantly paying a certain metabolic cost merely to stay alive...thus, in order to determine the actual metabolic cost of any particular activity, we must first subtract the basic metabolic cost from the total metabolic cost, any resulting difference then being the metabolic cost of that activity.

If, for example, an individual's basic metabolic cost while resting was 100 units per minute...and if his total metabolic cost increased to 150 units per minute while walking slowly on level ground...then the metabolic cost of walking at that pace under those conditions was 50 units per minute.

Unfortunately, when attempts have been made to determine the metabolic cost of positive work as compared to the metabolic cost of negative work, it appears that the basic metabolic cost was not subtracted from the totals. Instead, the meaningful comparison, the net metabolic costs, should have been compared.

At this point in time, I do not know just what the exact results of careful tests on this subject will be...but it appears that many of the tests conducted in the past, left a great deal to be desired, and that the conclusions based on those tests are in error.

People who are interested in meaningful areas of research in the broad field of exercise physiology might find it very fruitful to conduct careful tests in connection with the points raised in this chapter; in the meantime, we are conducting our own tests...which will be published in due course.

When and if it becomes possible to compare the metabolic cost of negative work with that of positive work on the basis of a meaningful standard, it may well be shown that the metabolic cost is in fact exactly the same in both cases; but even if not, it will certainly be shown that the difference, if any, is far less than it is now generally assumed to be.

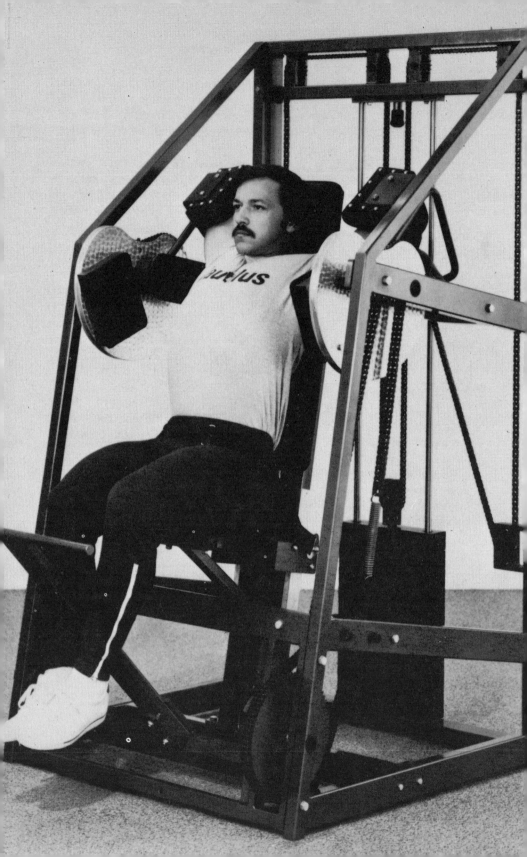

12
Flexibility and Metabolic Condition

By Arthur Jones

Let us discuss flexibility first as a result of strength training. The stereotype still exists in the minds of most people...bulging muscles are equated with a stiff, slow, and probably clumsy individual. In fact, the size of a man's muscles has very little or nothing to do with his actual flexibility.

It is certainly true that some individuals with large muscles do lack a normal degree of flexibility...it is also true that large muscles can be developed while doing absolutely nothing in the way of improving flexibility...and, in some rather rare cases, it is even true that the activities which built the large muscles also produced a loss of flexibility. But in the vast majority of cases, the size of the muscles has very little relationship to the existing degree of flexibility.

A trainee can build large, strong muscles while doing nothing for flexibility...or he can develop his muscles in a haphazard fashion and perhaps even reduce his flexibility...but he can, and he should, build his muscles and increase his flexibility at the same time, producing both favorable results from exactly the same exercises.

It must be clearly understood that the strength of the muscles is the only really productive factor involved in functional ability...an exerciser's muscles produce movement...his muscles perform work...his muscles are his only source of power for any purpose. In effect, and in fact, the muscles are the engine of the body. Without the strength of the muscles an individual would be utterly helpless, literally unable to move.

However, in the face of the previous clear and undeniable statement, it still remains true that an enormous number of coaches and athletes remain almost literally afraid of their muscles. Failing to understand the simple cause and effect relationships involved, or still believing a number of thoroughly disproved myths, they look upon the development of muscular strength as something to be avoided.

Functional ability is a result of at least five separate factors...1) muscular strength...2) neurological ability, which is genetically determined and not subject to improvement...3) bodily proportions, which are also genetically determined and not subject to improvement...4) cardiovascular ability...and 5) skill.

To that list of factors we can, and probably should, add flexibility...which, to at least some degree, is also genetically determined; but only to the extent that the absolute maximum possible ranges of movement are limited genetically. This simply means that some people have a greater potential for flexibility...some people can be extremely flexible, and some cannot.

Considered logically, it is immediately obvious that only one of those six factors is actually *productive*...superior neurological ability is an enormous advantage to an athlete, but only because it permits him to use his muscles in a more efficient manner; in effect, his muscles are given an advantage denied average men, but it is still the muscles that perform the work.

Ideal bodily proportions for a particular activity bestow another great advantage upon an athlete so blessed...but only because the result provides his muscles with an advantage leverage for his individual sport; and again, it is obvious that the muscles actually perform the work.

Adequate cardiovascular ability is another requirement...but no amount or level of cardiovascular endurance will produce movement; again, it is the muscles that perform the work.

Skill is also important, and can easily be the only difference between a champion and a clod...but only because the possession of a particular skill enables an athlete to use the strength of his muscles to the greatest possible advantage. And again, it is the muscles, and only the muscles, that perform the work.

If we add flexibility to this list, as we probably should...then it is again obvious that we still have only one productive factor; flexibility does not produce movement...instead, it permits movement. Only the muscles produce movement.

Of a list of six factors that determine functional ability, we have two that are not subject to improvement, neurological ability and bodily proportions...and we have four factors that are subject to improvement, 1) muscular strength, 2) cardiovascular ability, 3) skill, and 4) flexibility.

And, of the same list of six factors, we have only one factor that is actually productive...all of the factors are supportive in nature; they are certainly important, but only in the sense that they serve to support or improve the efficiency of the working muscles. These factors give the working muscles an

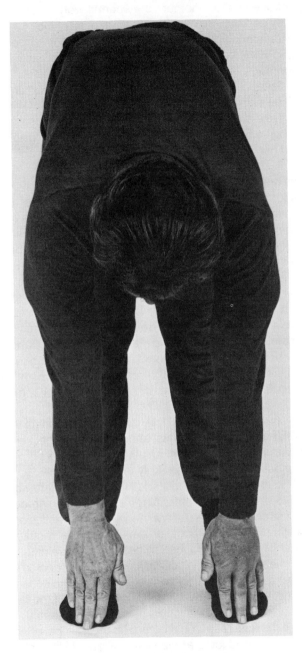

In the vast majority of cases, the size of an individual's muscles has very little relationship to the existing degree of flexibility.

advantage of one kind or another...they permit work, assist work, improve **work**; but, they certainly do not perform work of any kind.

Almost all outstanding athletes are blessed with both superior neurological ability and ideal bodily proportions for a particular activity...these two factors are primarily responsible for their success. When the factors of adequate cardiovascular ability, great skill, and the required degree of flexibiity for the individual sport are added, the result is a level of functional ability far above average...even when the strength of the muscles is only average. But the same man, given the same advantages, would be better at any activity if his muscles were also better than average and stronger than average.

In the vast majority of cases, however, it is almost impossible to convince such a man (or his coach) that increasing the strength of his muscles will improve his performance. On the contrary, in most cases, the athlete and his coach are both convinced that any increase in muscular size or strength would somehow hurt his performance. They utterly fail to understand the simple cause and effect relationships that determine functional ability. Such people are literally afraid to disturb a situation that appears good...little realizing that the really outstanding athlete has far more to gain from proper strength training than an average man does.

If they make any use of strength training at all, they usually confine it to their poorer athletes...being afraid to make the slightest change in their better athletes, for fear of disturbing some apparently mysterious factor. Then they try to justify this attitude on the grounds that strength training might make a particular athlete slower, less flexible, clumsy or somehow destroy his skill.

Hogwash...pure unadulterated hogwash. Proper strength training will improve any athlete, in any activity just short of playing checkers. The simple truth of the matter is that the better an athlete is, the more flexible, more enduring at any activity, and far less likely to suffer injury.

Sometime in the probably far distance future, all athletes in all sports will engage in two distinct types of training...strength training designed to improve overall strength and flexibility in general, and practice of a specialized sporting activity for the purpose of developing the required skills. Cardiovascular ability will be produced by both types of training.

But, in the meantime, millions of athletes are being denied the benefits of strength training simply and only because they and their coaches fail to understand the actual factors involved...to say nothing of the fact that literally thousands of injuries occur that could have been prevented.

During an extensive research program on the multiple effects of strength training, a project conducted at the United States Military Academy in the spring of 1975, careful tests were given for the purpose of determining the results that would be produced in the area of flexibility. Results? These showed an enormous increase in every area of flexibility, a direct result of the same strength training program that also produced an average strength increase of approximately 60 percent within an elapsed training time of only six weeks.

For purposes of comparing the results of the strength training program to the results produced by a normal football program of spring training, two groups of athetes were used...the first group called the Wholebody Group because they were trained in an overall fashion, consisted of 18 members of the West Point varsity football team...the second group, called the Control Group, consisted of 16 members of the same football squad that did not take part in the special training program.

Both groups were tested both before the training program and again six weeks later, at the end of the program. And both groups were involved in spring football practice during the period of the training program; thus, any differences in flexibility that showed up between the two groups could be attributed to the strength training program.

In the first test, trunk extension, the members of the Wholebody Group increased their range of movement an average of 7.22 inches...as compared to an average of only 0.62 inches for the Control Group. So, the subjects that were involved in the strength training program increased their flexibility by more than ten times as much as the other group did from football training.

In the second test, trunk flexion, the Wholebody Group increased an average of 2.67 inches...as compared to an improvement of 0.13 for the Control Group. Therefore, in this instance, the improvement for the strength trained athletes was more than twenty times as great as for the others.

In the third test, shoulder flexion, the Wholebody Group improved an average of 5.50 inches...compared to 0.50 inches for the Control Group. Again the strength trained group improved more than ten times as much as the other group.

A fourth test was also conducted, shoulder rotation, but the results of this test were not available at the time this chapter was written. This test involves the use of a pullover machine, a gonimeter, and motion pictures were made during both the before and after testing. While it was obvious at the time of testing that large scale increases were produced, the exact figures are not yet available.

Such dramatic improvements in flexibility are certainly not an accidental result of strength training...on the contrary, they are the carefully calculated tests that were produced by a properly designed program of full-range exercises; exercises capable of providing all of the requirements necessary to increase flexibility.

Flexibility is a result of stretching...pure and simple. No other factor is involved; but stretching is possible only under certain conditions, and stretching is not provided by most exercises performed for the purpose of increasing strength.

Stretching is a result of a movement that actually exceeds the momentarily existing range of possible movement...but such a range of movement alone is not enough; additionally there must be a force tending to pull the subject into the stretched position.

In effect, a subject cannot simply move into a stretched position...instead, he must be forced into a stretched position, pulled into it or pushed into it by a source of resistance that provides the required force. But he absolutely should not be forced into a stretched position suddenly; the result of such sudden movement may well be a pulled muscle instead of increased flexibility. Instead, he should steadily increase his ranges of possible movement through the use of gradually increasing resistance...thus, as his strength increases and he is able to use more weight, he will also be pulled or pushed into positions that were previously impossible.

However, producing increases in flexibility is one thing...and testing increases in flexibility is something else. So, for the purpose of testing, we did not utilize any resistance at all in the first three tests; instead, the results were determined simply by having the subjects move throughout as great a range of movement as possible without any outside source of force to assist them.

And in the fourth test, shoulder rotation, we used a constant amount of added resistance...40 pounds of weight were used during both before and after testing; if more weight had been used during the latter test, then additional force would have biased the results.

A great deal has been written recently on the subject of *negative work* as a factor in exercise, both pro and con...but it should be clearly understood that negative work is an absolute requirement for the purpose of increasing flexibility. It is negative work which provides the back pressure of force that is required to pull a subject into a stretched position; so, if negative work (or eccentric contractions) is removed from his exercises, any chance to improve flexibility has also been removed.

But even some exercises that involve negative work still fail to provide stretching, so even these exercises do absolutely nothing for flexibility; chinning exercises (or pull-ups), for example, may appear to stretch the muscle and connective tissues in the area of the shoulders...but in fact, a far greater range of possible movement in that area of the body is untouched in such exercises...simply because there is no force in the proper direction to force the involved body parts into an actually stretched position.

Dipping exercises (parallel dips), however, do provide good stretching in the opposite direction...provided there is enough resistance to force the body into a low enough position. This can be achieved best by performing dipping exercises in a *negative-only* fashion...by performing only the eccentric part of the movement with the muscles of the arms and chest; since such a style of training permits the subject to use far more resistance, a heavier weight will pull him into the stretched position.

It is obvious that a properly conducted program of stretch exercises can and should increase both strength and flexibility...and it will if the subject confines his attention to truly full-range exercises, and if he is careful in the arrangement of his overall program so that equal attention is given to the muscles on both sides of all joints.

And if the subject will get it out of his head that his muscles are something to be feared and thus neglected, training the muscles properly can only improve his performance...neglecting them can only hurt his performances and greatly increase his chances of injury.

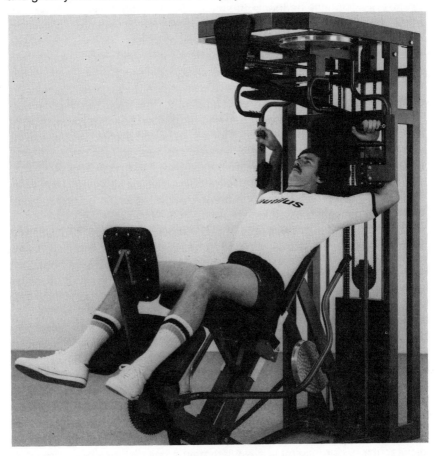

In effect, a subject cannot simply move into a stretched position...instead, he must be forced into a stretched position; pulled into it or pushed into it by a source of resistance that provides the required force.

Metabolic Condition

Contrary to widespread opinion, it now appears that there are three separate levels of condition...1) muscular strength...2) cardiovascular ability...and 3) a previously mentioned unsuspected level of condition that I have named *metabolic condition.*

Muscular strength can be built to a very high level with little or no improvement in cardiovascular ability. And it is well established that the exercises and activities that have traditionally been used for the improvement of cardiovascular condition will do almost nothing in the way of increasing muscular strength; in fact, it frequently happens that cardiovascular training actually produces a loss in muscular strength.

Thus, it frequently happens that a particular athlete has only one or the other...either strength or cardiovascular endurance, but not both. It is almost certain that two distinct types of training have been used; one type of exercise for the development of strength, and an entirely different type of activity for the development of cardiovascular ability.

Yet even when an athlete does have both strength and cardiovascular endurance, something of very great value is still missing...the third level of condition, the previously mentioned metabolic condition, is missing. As a result, the athlete can work very hard for a brief period of time...or, instead, he can work at a much lower level of intensity for a prolonged period of time. But he can not work with maximum intensity for a long period of time.

In effect, he can engage in brief anaerobic activities with a very high intensity of effort...or he could perform aerobic activities with a greatly reduced level of intensity for a much longer period of time.

At first glance it might well appear to be literally impossible to expect anything more from an athlete; after all, a muscle certainly cannot work with maximum intensity for much more than approximately one minute...and even then, the output will rapidly decline during the activity, simply because the athlete will be exhausting the working muscle fibers much faster than the resting fibers can recover.

In order to perform aerobic work (steady-state work) it is necessary to limit the level of intensity...the percentage of simultaneously working fibers must not be too high. An athlete must always have enough resting fibers ready to take over and continue the work as they are needed. If the percentage of working fibers is too high, it is simply impossible for the resting fibers to recover rapidly enough to take over the work as quickly as they are required.

When the unavoidable implications of the previous two paragraphs are understood, it then seems logical to assume that muscular strength and cardiovascular endurance must always remain some distance apart...must always be developed by separate and greatly divergent types of exercise. The real facts indicate otherwise.

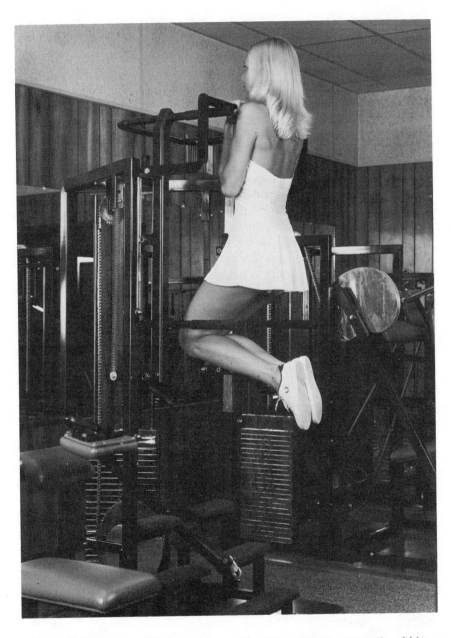

In order to produce significant increases in muscular strength within a reasonable period of time, the muscles must be trained as hard as possible...must be worked to a point of failure within a rather limited number of repetitions and over a short span of time.

Flexibility and Metabolic Condition

In the supervised research program in cooperation with the physical education staff of the United States Military Academy at West Point, New York, more than 100 military cadets were used as test subjects. To the best of our knowledge, this was the largest, most comprehensive, most carefully conducted, and probably the most extensive research program ever conducted in the area of strength training. In due course, a book will be published on the subject of this research project; but in this chapter I am limiting my remarks to one small but very important aspect of training that was clearly demonstrated during the West Point project.

During this project we were interested in all aspects of condition...we wanted to increase muscular strength as much as possible, and as quickly as possible...but we also wanted to produce large scale increases in cardiovascular condition...and we wished to demonstrate that both results could be produced by exactly the same style of training.

In a period of less than six weeks a group of 19 football players increased their strength by an average of approximately 60 percent...that's right, 60 percent, an average increase of 10 percent per week, a rate of strength increase previously considered to be literally impossible by most experts. And it must be clearly understood that these test subjects were not average subjects; instead, they were highly conditioned football players who were already quite strong at the beginning of the special training program; subjects with an average height of just below 6 feet, 2 inches, and an average weight well in excess of 200 pounds.

Producing such an almost unbelievable strength increase in such a short period of time would certainly have been a significant result even if absolutely nothing was accomplished in the way of cardiovascular improvement; but, in fact, an equally significant improvement in cardiovascular endurance was produced simultaneously...produced as a result of the same very brief training program that produced the spectacular strength increases.

Therefore, it appears that many of the experts have been wrong; in fact, it is neither necessary nor even desirable to conduct two distinct types of exercise programs, one program to produce strength increases and a second program to improve cardiovascular condition. In practice, it is easily possible to produce both results from the same program.

And, in order to produce the third level of condition, the previously mentioned metabolic condition, it is absolutely necessary to train in this fashion. It is necessary to train in a fashion that will unavoidably produce rapid and large scale increases in strength, in cardiovascular condition, and in metabolic condition.

And just what is metabolic condition? It is the ability to work at a high level of intensity for a prolonged period of time...the ability to work at a level very close to 100 percent of intensity for a period of at least 20 minutes, instead of one minute previously considered possible.

Work the muscles that hard for that period of time? No, that is impossible; but, it is possible to work the overall body that hard for that period of time...or, at least, it is possible if the subject has been trained properly. Proper style of training is the subject of this chapter.

In order to produce significant increases in muscular strength within a reasonable period of time, the muscles must be trained as hard as possible...must be worked to a point of failure within a rather limited number of repetitions and over a short span of time. In practice, best results seem to be produced when an exercise is performed for at least seven but not more than twelve repetitions...and when the exercise is continued to the point where it becomes literally impossible to perform another repetition in good form, continued to the point where 100 percent of momentarily available muscular strength is no longer capable of moving the resistance through a complete range of possible movement without a sacrifice of form.

Obviously, if such an intensity of work is employed, it is impossible to do more than one set of an exercise without a rest period between sets; thus, traditionally, the practice has been to perform one set of an exercise, then rest for three or four minutes in order to give the momentarily exhausted muscles time to recover their strength, and then perform a second set of the same exercise, then rest again, and so on. Such training will eventually build great strength, although it is not the best or fastest way even for the purpose of increasing strength; but, it will do very little in the way of improving cardiovascular condition.

Cardiovascular benefits will not result from such training for obvious reasons...1) because the pulse rate and the level of breathing will never be brought to a very high level...and 2) because the brief periods of hard work will be spaced with rather prolonged periods of total rest (between sets) that will permit the pulse rate and level of breathing to drop before additional work is started.

Cardiovascular benefits seem to be produced best when the pulse rate and the breathing rate are both raised to a high level...and are maintained at a high level for a prolonged period of time, 10 minutes, 15 minutes or even longer. Just how long such levels need to be maintained for the production of maximum cardiovascular benefits is a question that has not been satisfactorily answered; but, a period of 15 to 20 minutes will certainly produce large scale cardiovascular benefits even when such training is repeated only three times weekly.

Metabolic condition is the ability to work at a high level of intensity for a prolonged period of time...the ability to work at a level very close to 100 percent of intensity for a period of at least 20 minutes, instead of one minute previously considered possible.

Flexibility and Metabolic Condition

During the West Point project the subjects were trained only three times weekly...only one set of each exercise was performed during each work-out...every exercise was continued to a point of momentary muscular failure within a limited number of repetitions, seven to twelve repetitions. Very little in the way of rest was permitted between exercises, the minimum amount necessary to prevent cardiovascular failure...and the total elapsed training time during each workout varied from as little as 14 minutes to a bit more than 30 minutes.

If such a workout is conducted too fast at first...fast in the sense that little or no rest at all is permitted between exercises, then the subject will literally go into shock and be unable to continue...not because his muscles have been required to do something impossible...and not because he has ex-ceeded his cardiovascular ability in the normal meaning of the term...but ap-parently, because he lacks the metabolic ability to continue. At this point in time I do not know exactly why a subject fails under these conditions...but, obviously, such a failure clearly indicates that the subject is asking his body to perform something that is momentarily impossible.

If, for example, we work a starting trainee to a point of failure on a hip and back machine, immediately work him to a point of failure on a leg extension machine...we can reasonably expect him to quickly reach a point where he simply cannot continue, a point where he starts to show obvious signs of im-pending shock, which would be followed by total collapse if he was forced to continue working.

And yet, this collapse would occur at a point where neither his muscles nor his cardiovascular ability has been exceeded...the muscles we are ask-ing to work are rested fresh, and able to perform...the pulse rate is well with-in safe limits...the rate of breathing is within reasonable limits; but, the sub-ject cannot continue and will go into outright shock if forced to continue.

Just what is lacking? I do not really know, but it is obvious that a demand is being made that the body cannot meet.

If there is interest in totally unsupported theories, then I do have a theory...a theory that I have no great confidence in at this point in time; I think that the body may simply be unable to provide the required chemical changes that are necessary to work that hard for a prolonged period of time. The required oxygen is available, and the circulatory system is capable of distributing it rapidly enough...the required nutrients are also available, but perhaps the body cannot provide the required metabolic changes at such a pace.

In any case, regardless of the actual cause and effect situation involved, the results are obvious...the subject simply cannot continue to work.

Therefore, at the start of such a training program, a brief amount of rest must be permitted between exercises...not much rest, but some rest, perhaps one to two minutes, depending upon the individual trainee.

124

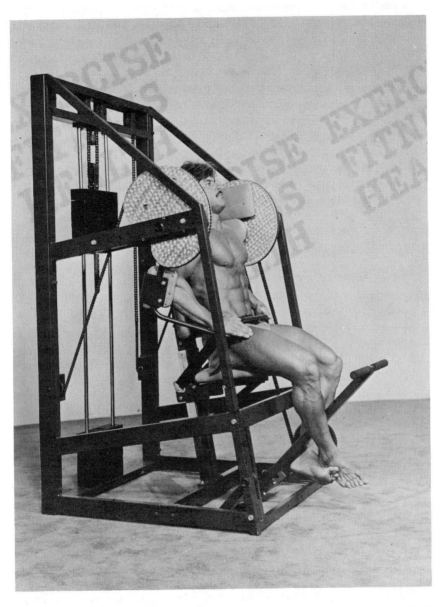

It is obvious that a properly conducted program of strength exercises can and should increase both strength and flexibility...and it will if the subject confines his attention to truly full-range exercises, and if he is careful in the arrangement of his overall program so that equal attention is given to the muscles on both sides of all joints.

However, as training continues from week to week, the pace of the training should be increased...so that, after approximately four weeks, little or no rest is permitted between exercises. By that point in the training program the subjects should move from one exercise to the next exercise as rapidly as possible, with very little rest between exercises.

Now, bear in mind that a fast pace of training certainly does not mean that the exercise movements themselves are performed rapidly...on the contrary, the movements should be fairly slow and perfectly smooth with absolutely nothing in the way of sudden movement or jerking. A fast pace of training simply means that no rest is permitted between exercises.

Once a subject becomes capable of training in this fashion without going into shock as a result, then it becomes possible to work his muscles to a point of momentary failure while maintaining both the pulse rate and breathing at very high levels throughout the entire workout. And, since it was impossible for the beginning trainee to work in this fashion, it is thus obvious that something besides strength and cardiovascular ability has been improved...the subject has also greatly improved his metabolic ability.

And just what advantage does such a factor give an athlete? Well, how would a coach like to have a football team that literally did not require rest for a period of 30 minutes? Such a team could return to scrimmage immediately without the necessity to huddle...thus giving their opponents no chance to rest.

As an example of just how big a factor this can be, I will cite one example, a typical example from our experience at West Point. During his seventh workout, this subject required 24 minutes for his workout...but less than six weeks later, during his twenty-first workout, he performed an identical workout in only 18 minutes even though he was then using approximately 60 percent more resistance for the same number of repetitions.

His workout length was reduced by 25 percent, while his level of resistance was increased by 60 percent...thus his rate of work per minute was increased by more than 100 percent, more than double. Instead of doing 100 units of work in 24 minutes, or 4.1 units of work per minute, he was doing 160 units of work in 18 mninutes, or 8.8 units of work per minute.

And he worked at a more than doubled rate while showing a far lower pulse rate...during the seventh workout his pulse rate was in excess of 200, but during the twenty-first workout his pulse rate was always below 180.

Also, at the end of his seventh workout, the subject was near a point of collapse, and it took him several hours to return to a normal condition...whereas, at the end of the twenty-first workout, the subject had improved his recovery ability to such an extent that he literally could have repeated the workout after a rest of about 10 minutes.

His strength was greatly improved, and his capacity for work was also greatly improved...but just what effect was produced in regard to cardiovascular ability?

Significant improvement was demonstrated on all 60 separate tests conducted for the purpose of determining cardiovascular improvements. For example, the subjects we trained improved their time in the two mile run by an average of 88 seconds in a period of six weeks; as compared to an improvement of only 20 seconds produced by a control group of matched subjects that were not trained in this fashion. Both groups were involved in spring football training.

Much more detailed accounts of this style of training will be published at a later date, and in the meantime several other large scale projects are being conducted in an effort to determine the exact results of such training; but it must be clearly understood that this style of training is of such a high intensity that very little of it is either necessary or desirable. Do not make the mistake of assuming that longer or more frequent workouts of this kind will produce even better results. On the contrary, brief training is far more than a possibility...it is an outright requirement for good results.

It is almost inevitable that at least some *experts* will immediately jump to a hasty conclusion; whereupon, they will rush into print to deny that anything new is involved. But I hereby warn them clearly in advance that the effects and results I am concerned with here apparently are new...and while I certainly do not even pretend to understand all of the biological factors involved, I am at least aware of the obvious cause and effect.

The West Point project was not the first example of such a style of training...on the contrary, we have been training a large number of subjects in this fashion for the last several years in Florida and elsewhere. More than 400 individual workouts were conducted at too fast a pace. One subject was forced to stop near the middle of one of his workouts...forced to stop because I was trying to train him at a pace that he could not maintain.

But all of the other subjects finished all of their workouts, and even that one subject finished all of his other workouts; although, I am certain that many of them did not believe at the time that they would finish, and equally certain that most of the subjects would never have pushed themselves at the necessary pace if left to their own devices.

Such training requires close and informed supervision...close supervision to assure that the pace is fast enough, and informed (or at least experienced) supervision to assure that the pace is not too fast. The workout absolutely must not be permitted to degenerate into a race against the clock...each and every exercise must be performed properly, the exercise movements should be fairly slow, and the exercise must be continued until an actual point of muscular failure is reached; if not, then a large part of the potential strength benefits will not be produced.

Nearly four years ago, one would-be *expert* from another state visited our facilities in Florida for the purpose, he said, of evaluating our equipment and style of training. He spent two weeks here, but refused to follow instructions. Later, he remarked that the training did not make him sick, that he could see nothing different about it. Well, obviously, the purpose of training is not to make the subject sick, and we had gone to great lengths with this man in successful efforts to keep from making him sick...which efforts, in that case, were worse than wasted, since he learned absolutely nothing from the experience.

Properly conducted, such training will not make the subjects sick...but it can, and it will, if the subjects are pushed too hard at first. And while I am perfectly aware that several other styles and types of training will sometimes produce an apparently similar reaction, I repeat that there is a distinct, if not yet fully understood, difference.

And I am also clearly aware that there is another difference of far greater importance...the third level of condition, metabolic condition, as I mean the term, apparently cannot be produced by any other style of training. An athlete trained properly in this fashion will still be going strong in any activity requiring prolonged, heavy exertion for a long period of time after his opponent is stretched out in a state of outright collapse.

This type of training would probably be of little or no value for a weight lifter, or a shot putter...but it is the best type of training by far for a football player, a basketball player, a wrestler, a soccer player, a swimmer or a person involved in any other activity requiring both strength and cardiovascular endurance.

13
Predicting Athletic Ability

By Arthur Jones

Playing basketball certainly will not make you seven feet tall...and no amount of exercise will transform a genetically inferior specimen into an outstanding athlete, and neither will anything else.

People are not born equal; the potential for physical development varies enormously...and while it is true that properly performed exercise will greatly improve the functional ability of almost literally anybody, it is also true that the final results will not be equal.

Proper exercise, like anything else, has certain basic requirements...if these requirements are provided, then the results will be good; if not, then the results will be poor...it's just that simple. But what are the requirements for proper exercise? What should we do? What should we avoid?

The claims and counterclaims now being made in the field of exercise have produced far more confusion than understanding...whom to believe?...what to believe? This is unfortunate, because the demonstrated benefits of properly conducted exercise are of enormous value.

To begin with, we must clearly understand the limitations of exercise...what it can do, and what it cannot do. And we must also understand the individual limitations of people; in effect, who can and who can't.

Contrary to popular opinion, exercise does not produce physical changes of any sort...instead, exercise stimulates physical changes. This statement is neither a play on words nor a point to be considered lightly.

Physical changes are produced by the body itself...in response to a demonstrated need for such changes. Exercise provides the stimulation for these changes by imposing an overload of some sort on the body, by asking the body to perform at a level beyond its existing functional ability.

Exercise that does not involve an overload of some sort is utterly worthless for the purpose of improving functional ability; so, the results of exercise are in proportion to the quality of the exercise performed, rather than the quantity. In exercise, at least, more is certainly not better, and is usually worse.

Secondly...exercise cannot change your genetic potential; your potential for physical improvement was genetically determined before birth. So, there is a limit to possible physical improvement, a limit that varies widely on an individual basis.

A large part of the presently existing confusion in the field of exercise is a direct result of a general failure to understand the above point...or an unwillingness to accept it. Having seen the results that somebody else produced by exercise, many people are almost desperately seeking the secret to similar results. Such people will try almost literally anything that is suggested.

The potential for physical improvement varies enormously. Although it can't be measured with a very high degree of accuracy, it is now possible to anticipate the limits of physical development...a bit later we will cover the procedures required for making such determinations. The purpose of this series of chapters can thus be divided into two parts...first, a detailed coverage of the measurement and testing procedures required for a practical evaluation of the several physiological factors that contribute to functional ability...and, secondly, a step-by-step outline of the methods required for improving some of these factors.

In very simple terms...first we will tell you what you can do...and then we will tell you how to do it. And, along the way, we will tell you several things that you cannot do...as well as a number of things that you should not do.

The ability to perform any physical activity is determined by at least six factors, all of which are important. Some of these factors are subject to improvement, and some are not. These factors are...one, bodily proportions...two, cardiovascular ability...three, flexibility...four, muscular strength ...five, neurological ability..and, six, skill.

Exercise will do absolutely nothing to improve your bodily proportions...and will probably do nothing to improve your neurological ability; the first of these factors is certainly determined by genetics...the second is probably determined by genetics. So, in effect, we are stuck with what we have in these areas, good or bad.

Skill is a result of practice...practice devoted to a particular activity, practice involving specificity; thus it follows that properly conducted exercise will produce absolutely nothing in the way of an increase in skill.

Why?

Because proper exercise involves an overload...and because proper skill training involves total specificity; factors that are mutually exclusive...if you have one, then you obviously cannot have the other.

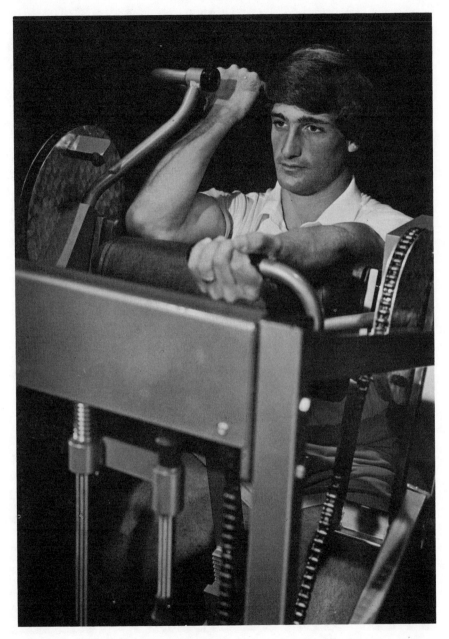

Proper exercise, like anything else, has certain basic requirements...if these requirements are provided, then the results will be good; if not, then the results will be poor...it's just that simple.

Thus, exercise will not help your skill, but improperly performed exercise may hurt your skill; so, do not make the mistake of confusing exercise, which is performed for the purpose of improving your physiological functional ability...and practice, which is performed for the purpose of improving your skill.

Specificity in exercise is utterly impossible, an outright myth; and anything approaching specificity in exercise is a terrible mistake, because it will do little or nothing in the way of improving the physiological factors involved in performance...but it certainly will hurt your skill.

Thus, three of the six factors cannot be helped by exercise...we cannot improve our bodily proportions...we cannot increase our neurological ability...and we cannot help our skill by exercise.

But, we certainly can increase our muscular strength...we can improve our cardiovascular ability...and we can increase our flexibility; all three of which factors are important for functional ability in any activity...and the only possible way to improve any of these factors is exercise.

So, exercise is important, far more important than most people even suspect; yet it still remains true that most of the time and energy devoted to exercise is utterly wasted...or worse, since poorly performed exercise is actually counterproductive.

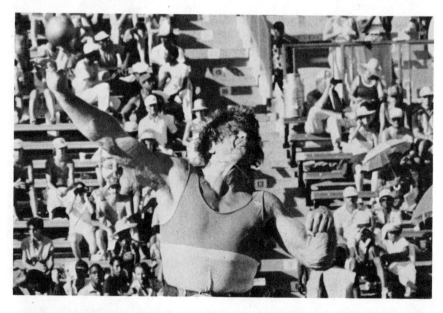

...Because proper exercise involves an overload...and because proper skill training involves total specificity factors that are mutually exclusive...if you have one, then you obviously cannot have the other.

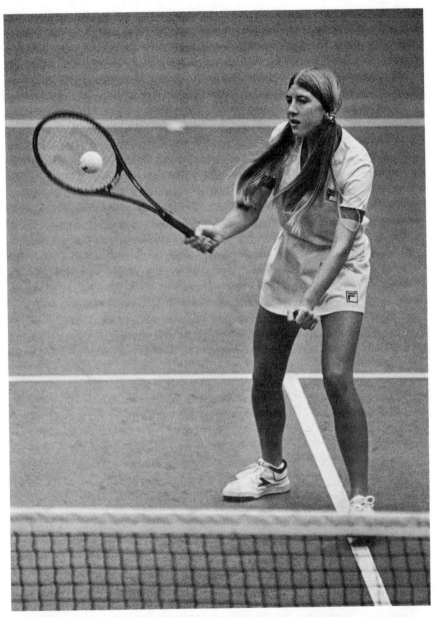

The most common failing in today's athletes exists in the area of muscular strength...which is ironic, to say the least; because muscular strength can almost always be increased to a signifiant degree...and doing so will increase the functional ability of any athlete, in any sport.

This remains true for two reasons...primarily because most people do not undertand the very simple cause and effect relationships involved in exercise...and, secondly, because many people are still trying to produce results that are simply impossible.

A large part of the confusion that currently exists on the subject of exercise is a direct result of the fact that functional ability is a result of the several factors that I have listed previously...and while it is obvious that the ultimate level of performance in any activity will be reached only when all of the contributing factors are ideal, it still remains possible to reach a level of performance that is far above average even when one or more of the factors is not ideal.

Thus, it happens that many apparent exceptions can be seen in any sport; some athletes do not, for example, have the best bodily proportions for a particular activity...yet still manage to perform at or near a championship level.

But such an example proves literally nothing.,..the same individual, given ideal bodily proportions, would perform even better. In such cases, a weakness in one area is compensated for by advantage in another area; but regardless of his level of performance, such an individual is still being held back by his weakness in one area.

The most common failure in today's athletes exists in the area of muscular strength...which is ironic, to say the least because muscular strength can almost always be increased to a significant degree...and in doing so will increase the functional ability of any athlete, in any sport.

In general, today's athletes do not perform because they are strong; quite the contrary, most athletes perform well in spite of the fact that they are actually quite weak. Very few athletes in any sport are involved in any sort of meaningful strength training program...and, as mentioned earlier, most of the exercise that is performed is wasted, failing to produce the desired results.

A large part of this common failure to utilize meaningful strength training programs is due to the fact that many coaches are still afraid of strength training...which fear, in turn, stems from the fact that very few coaches really understand the role that muscular strength plays in physical performance.

Properly performed strength training will greatly increase an athlete's flexibiity...yet most coaches still remain convinced that increased muscular size and strength will somehow reduce the flexibility of their athletes. The old muscle bound myth lives on.

Increased muscular strength will also increase the speed of movement in any activity...yet many coaches still believe that increased strength will reduce the speed of their athletes.

In later articles, we will carefully examine all of the factors that contribute to functional ability...for the sake of clarity, these factors will be discussed one at a time. But it must be clearly understood that all of the factors are important, and it must be remembered that the relationship of factors is also important; that all of the factors work together to produce the final result.

And it must also be understood that a factor which provided an advantage in one activity could easily pose a problem in another activity; an ideal basketball player, for example, might be eight feet tall...while the same bodily proportions would be an utter disaster for a gymnast.

In the next chapter I will discuss the factor of great importance in any sport, and one that can easily be the only difference between a world champion and an outright failure. Just what is neurological ability? How does it contribute to athletic ability? Can it be measured, and if so, how? These and many other important questions on the subject of neurological ability will be covered in a simple, practical manner.

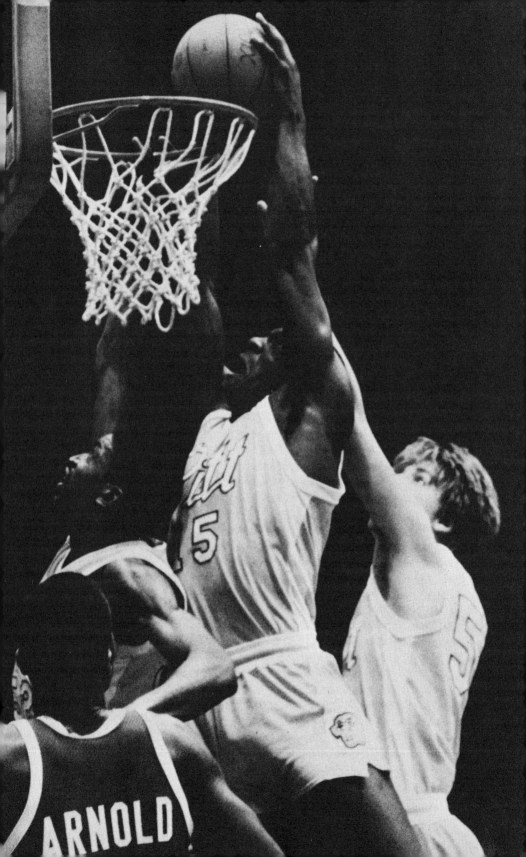

14
The Missing Link in Athletic Performance

By Arthur Jones

Human performance is a result of six factors, all of which are important...some of which are subject to improvement, while some are not.

These factors are in no particular order...one, cardiovascular ability...two, flexibility...three, skill...four, muscular strength...five, bodily proportions... and, six, neurological ability. All of the first four factors certainly can be improved by proper training...some form of exercise is being required to improve cardiovascular ability, flexibility and muscular strength...while skill is improved in only one way, by the proper application of skill training, by performance of the activity itself, with total specificity.

Exercise is one thing...while skill training is an entirely different matter; exercise is utterly worthless unless it involves an overload of some kind...but skill training literally must not involve an overload. Exercise must be hard, as hard as possible if good results are your goal...but skill training must not be hard, must not be continued to the point that it becomes exhausting.

So don't confuse the two entirely different types of training...and don't be misled into believing that any exercise is specific to a particular sport. Strength is general, flexibiity is general, cardiovascular ability is general...and all three of these important factors can and should be improved by the correct application of proper exercise...but skill is utterly specific and can be improved in only one way.

The fifth factor, bodily proportions cannot be improved...so you are stuck with what you have, good or bad. Proportions that are ideal for one sport may be utterly wrong for another activity...great height and long arms are certainly an advantage in basketball, but the same proportions would certainly ruin a gymnast. A particular athlete can obviously do nothing about his own bodily proportions...but a coach, by being aware of the importance of this factor, can and should recruit athletes with the proper bodily proportions for a given sport; and, to a large degree, this is already being done.

Which brings us to the last factor, neurological ability...a factor of great importance, but one that is not at all well known...the existence of which is not even suspected by most coaches and athletes. Not even suspected in spite of the fact that this one important factor can easily be the only difference between a world champion athlete and a complete failure...everything else being equal. Neurological ability has largely been ignored for at least three reasons...first, for the simple reason that most coaches, athletes, doctors and even exercise physiologists have never even heard of it...secondly, because most of the neurologists and neurosurgeons who were aware of this factor have assumed that it was an entirely genetic factor that was not subject to improvement; and thus, they tend to ignore a factor that can't be helped...and, finally, because there was no practical manner in which neurological ability could be measured.

Which immediately raises several interesting questions...one, just what is neurological ability?...two, how do we know it can't be improved?...and, three, how do we prove its very existence if we can't even measure it?

ONE...neurological ability is your abilty to stimulate muscular contraction. Muscular contraction is stimulated by your nerve, but it is utterly impossible to stimulate the contraction of all of the fibers in any muscle at the same time. If a muscle is rested, then all of the fibers could be contracted simultaneously if the nervous stimulation to the muscle were strong enough, which it is not.

The only possible way to stimulate simultaneous contraction of all of the fibers in a muscle is by electrocution. So, in effect and in fact, you can only use a small part of any muscle at any given time...even when you are straining in an all-out, maximum, do or die attempt, you are still only using a rather small part of your muscles, while most of your muscular fibers remain totally relaxed, contributing absolutely nothing to the work. But it does not follow that all people are equal in this regard. On the contrary, some people can obviously use a much larger than average percentage of their muscular fibers during a maximum effort. Such people are much stronger than average, for no apparent reason...such people have superior neurological ability.

TWO...it has been generally assumed that neurological ability was determined entirely by genetics; and if so, then obviously it cannot be improved...like bodily proportions, you are stuck with what you are born with, good or bad. But...until very recently, it has been impossible to measure neurological ability; so, we really have had no means of determing whether it could be improved or not. At this point in time (April, 1977), I still have no

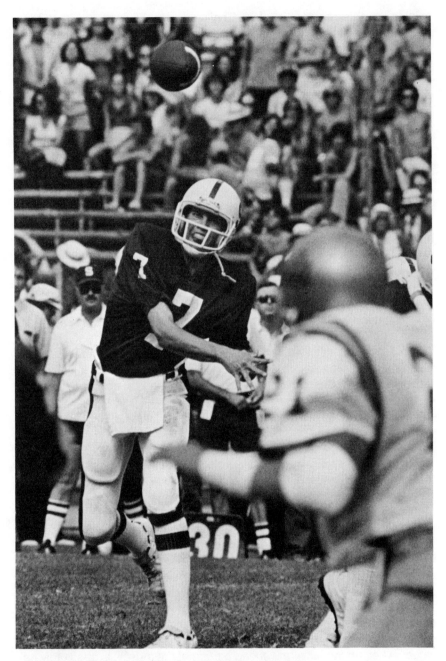

Human performance is a result of six factors, all of which are important...some of which are subject to improvement, while some are not.

opinion on this mattter. In plain English, I simply don't know whether neurological ability can be improved or not; but I do know that we now have a means of finding out for sure...because, finally, we do have a method for measuring neurological ability.

THREE...proving the very existence of variations in neurological ability was, until recently, a hit or miss proposition at best because we couldn't measure it. Yet such variations were obvious even if they couldn't be measured.

When all of the other factors were carefully considered, some people were far stronger than average, for no apparent reason...and when the same factors were considered in other cases, some people were much weaker than average. And when a stronger than average man was compared to a weaker than average man, it was immediately obvious that some unknown factor was responsibile for the great difference in strength...the only possible solution to this undeniable situation was that the stronger man was using a higher percentage of his muscle fibers; he was neurologically superior to the weaker man. His muscles were in no way better, his bodily proportions were in no way better, and since a true test of raw strength does not involve skill, it was also obvious that his skill was not responsible for the difference; so, the only difference rested on the fact that he was simply able to use a greater number of muscle fibers simultaneously.

That much, at least, I was aware of as long as twenty years ago...but, until recently, it was knowledge of little or no practical value; since we had no reasonably accurate method of measuring neurological ability, we couldn't do much in a practical sense with the information that we did have...but now we can; now we can measure it, and now we can put this information to use in a very important and practical manner. Like most things, the answer when I finally hit upon it, was utterly simple; so obvious that I literally felt like a fool for not realizing it years earlier..."Neurological ability is in inverse proportion to your anaerobic muscular endurance." This statement, at first glance, is a bit of a tongue twister...as well as being somewhat difficult to grasp immediately. But the following explanation will, I believe, make it very easy to understand...and will, secondly, make it obvious that this information can indeed be used in a very practical manner in all sports.

As mentioned earlier, it is utterly impossible to contract all of the fibers of any given muscle simultaneously...the result being that you are using only a small part of any muscle even when you are working as hard as possible.

Thus it is obvious that a very large part of a muscle, literally most of the muscle, is resting even when you are working as hard as possible. This might lead us to assume that this unworking part of the muscle is of no value...when, in fact, this unworking portion of the muscle is absolutely essential; because, without it, our muscular endurance would be almost zero.

If we could (which we cannot) contract all of the fibers in a muscle simultaneously, then we would certainly be strong...would be almost unbelievably strong; but we would have almost nothing in the way of muscular endurance because, if all of our fibers were working at the same time, then they would become exhausted at the same time, and all would be required to rest at the same time. So we would be very strong indeed...for one brief effort, after which effort we would be literally helpless, unable to move. On the other hand, if we could use only one percent of a muscle even during a maximum effort, then our strength would be very low...but our muscular endurance would be almost infinite.

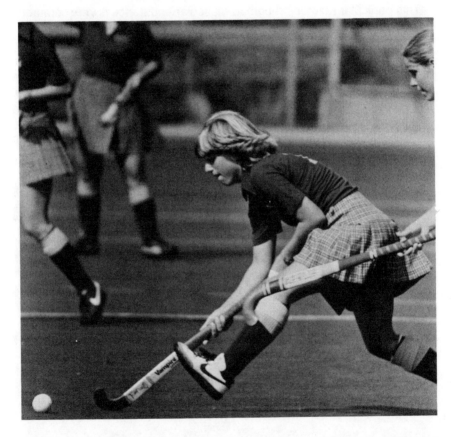

Exercise is one thing...while skill training is an entirely different matter; exercise is utterly worthless unless it involves an overload of some kind...but skill training literally must not involve an overload. Exercise must be hard, as hard as possible if good results are your goal...but skill training must not be hard, must not be continued to the point that it becomes exhausting.

The Missing Link in Athletic Performance

In my own case, I have known for more than thirty years that my strength and muscular endurance maintain a certain relationship...when my strength increases, then my muscular endurance also increases in exact proportion. Thus, when I can bench press 300 pounds once, I know that I can perform exactly ten repetitions with 250 pounds, and vice versa. When I can curl a 100 pound barbell ten times, then I know that I can curl a 120 pound barbell once, and vice versa. This ratio, for me, has remained absolutely constant for at least thirty years that I am aware of...I can perform one repetition with 20 percent more than I can use for ten repetitions. So, if I know my strength level, then I also know my level of muscular endurance...and, if I know my level of muscular endurance, then I know my strength level.

This particular ratio of strength to muscular endurance is very common, but it certainly does not apply to everybody. I have seen many exceptions in both directions; but, until recently, I failed to appreciate the significance of these exceptions. If, for example, three apparently identical triplets were tested, and if all three of them could bench press exactly 300 pounds during a maximum effort...but if, during an endurance test with 250 pounds, one man performed ten repetitions, while a second man failed after only four repetitions, and the third was able to perform fifteen repetitions...then who is the better athlete, at least insofar as neurological ability is concerned? And why is he better?

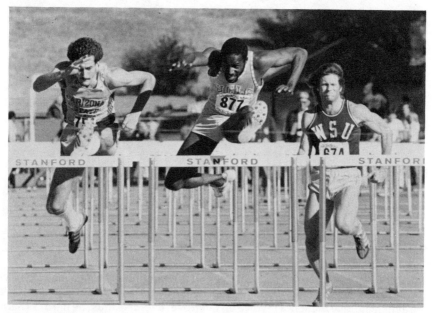

You are using only a small part of any muscle even when you are working as hard as possible.

Surprising as it may seem at first glance, the best man is the one who was able to perform the least number of repetitions. The man who failed after only four repetitions with 250 pounds has greater neurological ability than the man who did ten repetitions, and far greater ability than the man who performed fifteen repetitions.

The above example, for several reasons, is really not a valid test. To begin with, the bench press with a barbell involves far too much skill to be a valid test of pure strength...secondly, such a result would be impossible if the triplets really were identical, because the neurological superior man would be far stronger than the other two men if he had identical bodily proportions and muscular size.

So that example, while not perfectly valid, should be understood to be just what it is, an example intended to help make a point. If the triplets really were identical in every way except neurological ability, then the results would be somewhat as follows...the first man would bench press 300 pounds once, and then would perform ten repetitions with 250 pounds...the second man would bench press 450 pounds once, but would get only four repetitions with 375 pounds...while the third man would bench press only 200 pounds once, but would be able to get fifteen repetitions with 165 pounds.

In all three cases the men would be given approximately 83 percent of their best maximum lift. The man who got the least number of repetitions would be the better man, neurologically.

Why? Because, since he was using a higher than normal percentage of his total number of available muscle fibers, it obviously follows that his anaerobic muscular endurance would be lower. When the above information is fully digested, it then becomes possible to utilize this knowledge in a very valuable testing procedure for your athletes.

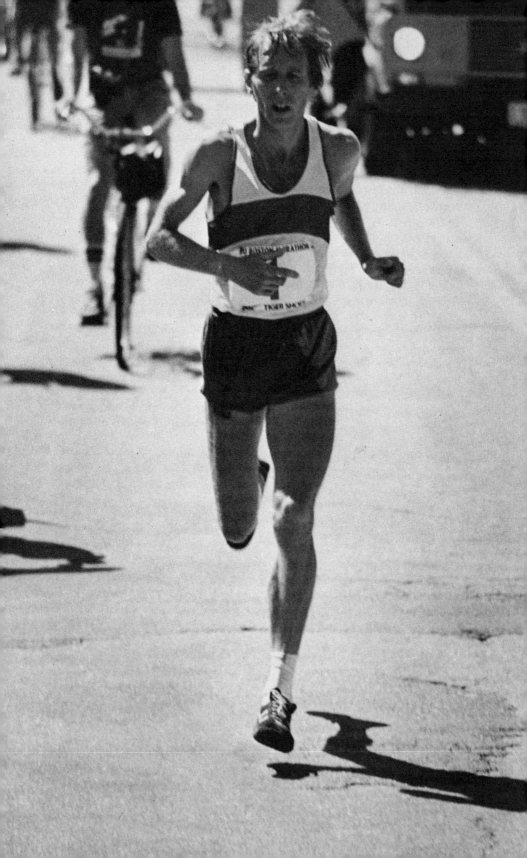

15
The Nervous System in Sports

By Arthur Jones

A clear understanding of a few simple facts about the nervous system is essential to an understanding of human performance. But do not be put off through a fear of medical terms or complex theory. The following is written in plain language...and the information presented is important to anybody involved in sports of any kind.

I want to make at least two points perfectly clear. First, it is impossible to involve the entire mass of any skeletal muscle in a normal contraction. This simply means that a person never uses more than a rather small percentage of any muscle at any point in time. Even in a maximum possible live or die attempt, only part of any muscle is being used...while the balance of the muscle, the largest part, is resting.

But if that is true, it might be asked, then what purpose does the extra unusable mass of muscle serve? The extra muscular mass serves a very important purpose, it provides muscular endurance. And it is usable, but not in concert with the rest of the muscle.

If all of the fibers in a muscle are fired simultaneously, the resulting force would be so great that the muscle would probably be torn loose from the bones. Or the bones themselves might be broken. Some people surviving accidental electrocution suffer broken bones as a direct result of the violent muscular contractions that are produced by a strong electrical shock; and electrocution almost always produces torn muscles or connective tissues.

The following figures and percentages are not intended to represent an exact situation; instead, they are merely used as a necessary part of an example, intended to make the previously mentioned point clear.

If, for example, a particular muscle contains a total of 100 fibers, a person might be able to contract only 30 of those fibers at any particular moment. Thus, even when he is working as hard as possible, he would be using only 30 percent of the available fibers...while 70 percent of the fibers were resting.

If a person could use 100 percent of a muscle simultaneously, and if he could withstand the resulting forces, then he would be utterly helpless after one very brief effort...because all of the fibers would be exhausted simultaneously, leaving absolutey nothing in reserve for a second effort.

Individual muscle fibers contract as hard as possible, all or nothing. So, in a maximum effort, some of the fibers are working as hard as possible, and some are doing nothing.

When a person reaches a point of momentary muscular failure, he may think that his strength has been totally exhausted; but in fact, a very high percentage of strength is still available. It simply is not enough to produce movement against the imposed resistance.

For example, if a person performs one repetition of a maximum bench press with 300 pounds, then it will be impossible to perform a second repetition immediately. But not because his momentary level of strength has suddenly been reduced to zero. In fact, his strength will be almost as high as it was at the start; but not quite high enough to lift the weight a second time.

Performing one maximum repetition reduces a person's beginning strength level by approximately 4 percent...leaving him with about 96 percent of his starting strength left to perform a truly maximum lift, and anything less will not do it. So the person is forced to stop, even though 96 percent of his strength is still available.

But, a person might say, if I use only 30 percent of a muscle, even in a maximum lift, then I should be able to perform several repetitions with a maximum weight; the first repetition would exhaust 30 percent of the muscle, the second repetition would exhaust a different 30 percent of the muscle, the third repetition would exhaust a final 30 percent of the muscle, and I would still have 10 percent of the muscle remaining unused.

This would be true...if the same fibers worked throughout the entire repetition; but they do not. The contraction of an individual muscle fiber is very brief; and in most situations, a fiber cannot continue to produce force throughout an entire movement. So individual fibers contract as hard as possible, but very briefly...and if force is still needed, then another fiber takes over and continues the work. If a person will observe a muscle during hard work, he can actually see the twitching that occurs during strong and continued muscular contraction.

So, if it is true that a muscle uses only 30 percent of its fibers during a maximum effort, then it is obvious that something less than 30 percent of the fibers are available immediately for a second effort.

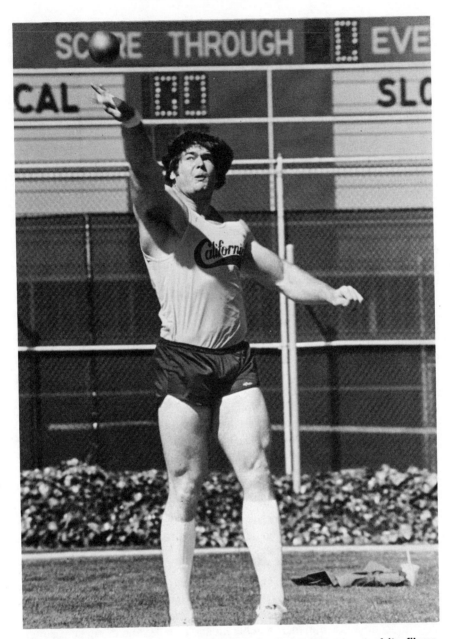

A fresh, rested muscle is capable of contracting 100 percent of its fibers simultaneously...but the nervous system is not. Muscular contraction is triggered by an electrical impulse from the nervous system, and there are not enough nerves available to stimulate all of the fibers at the same time.

A fresh, rested muscle is capable of contracting 100 percent of its fibers simultaneously...but the nervous system is not. Muscular contraction is triggered by an electrical impulse from the nervous system, and there are not enough nerves available to stimulate all of the fibers at the same time.

So, even when all of the nerves are working simultaneously, there are only enough nerves to trigger 30 percent of the total number of muscle fibers. Once triggered, a second repetition immediately following will be even weaker for two reasons. First, because then the individual will not have enough fresh fibers available to take advantage of the stimulation that is being provided...and, secondly, because the electrical stimulation from the nerves will also be weaker.

This leads to my second point. If an average man can contract only 30 percent of a particular muscle, it does not follow that all men are thus equal, some individuals can contract as much as 40 percent of the same muscle, and a few rare individuals can contract 50 percent of the muscle.

This means, in practical terms, that some men are far stronger than other men, all else being equal.

But it also means that these stronger-than-average men have less than an average amount of muscular endurance—not cardiovascular endurance, which has absolutely nothing to do with the matter, but muscular endurance.

If an average man, a 30 percenter, can bench press 300 pounds once, then he can perform ten repetitions with 250 pounds, and will fail while attempting an eleventh repetition.

But a smaller man with less muscular bulk might also bench press 300 pounds once...if his nervous system was better than average, if, for example, he was a 40 percenter. Yet this same man would not be able to perform 10 repetitions with 250 pounds; instead, he might fail after only 7 repetitions. His maximum strength would be equal to that of the larger man, but his muscular endurance would be less.

In fact, the bench press is actually not a very good lift to base such a comparison, simply because bench pressing is a test of skill as well as strength. But if a pure test of strength is used, then the results would be close to the percentages shown previously.

Such differences are genetically determined; which means, in plain language, that a person can do absolutely nothing to improve his nervous system. Most athletes are blessed with better than average nervous systems, which is largely responsible for the fact that they are athletes.

Almost anybody can increase his muscular bulk, and doing so will make him stronger; because 30 percent of a large muscle will produce more force than 30 percent of a small muscle. But it does not follow that all men can increase their strength equally, although the percentage of strength increase may be equal.

The Nervous System in Sports

Two men might be identical twins, with all visible factors including muscular bulk being exactly equal...the only difference being the fact that one man was average, a 30 percenter, while the other man was above average, a 40 percenter. In such a case, the 40 percenter would be markedly stronger, for no apparent reason; he would be stronger because he was able to use a large part of his total muscular bulk during a maximum effort.

His muscle would in no way be superior to the muscle of the other man. His greater strength would be a result of a better than average nervous system.

The weaker man might be able to bench press 150 pounds, while the stronger man could lift 200 pounds in the same manner; and then, later, as a result of strength training, the weaker man might double his strength, thus making it possible for him to bench press 300 pounds...while the stronger man would increase his strength by an equal percentage, but by a greater amount, and would then be able to bench press 400 pounds.

So the man with the weaker nervous system actually has more to gain from strength training than the average man does. This is simple once the related facts are clearly understood; but in many cases, this leads to confusion rather than understanding.

The result in many cases is that the very individuals who stand to gain the most from strength training are the onces who avoid it entirely.

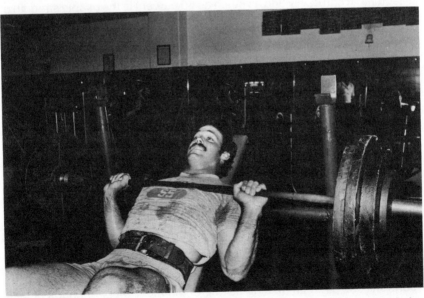

In practical terms, some men are far stronger than other men, all else being equal.

A man with only an average amount of muscular bulk, but a superior nervous system may well be stronger than another individual with much muscular bulk but with only an average nervous system. In this case it becomes easy to make the mistake of assuming that the extra muscular bulk is useless, or even that it somehow makes the man weaker.

Additional confusion is added by another common mistake; skill is often mistaken for strength...so a weaker man might be able to bench press more than a stronger man, if he is more skillful in the performance of that particular lift.

So if we have one man with great skill and a superior nervous system, then he might bench press far more weight than a much larger man with an average nervous system who has very little skill at bench pressing. In this case, it will appear that the greater muscular bulk is of no value, but such an appearance is utterly false.

A muscle is strong in almost direct proportion to its cross-sectional area; so the larger the muscle, the greater the strength. But a third factor now enters the picture to confuse the issue even more. Overall size is often mistaken for muscular size...a large arm may contain a high percentage of fat, and the actual muscular size may be only average. Fat will make a person larger, but fat is not muscle...fat does not contract, fat does not produce force, fat merely adds the burden of non-working weight.

And a fourth factor adds even more confusion. Bodily leverage is a genetic factor that can easily add as much as 50 percent to the usable strength of an individual. One man, with short arms, may lift a barbell a distance of only 14 inches in a bench press...while another man, with longer arms, may lift the barbell 21 inches in a bench press, 50 percent more than the other man.

Outstanding athletes usually have very good bodily leverage for a particular activity, a superior nervous system and great skill...but they almost never have more than average muscular bulk. Convincing such a man that he stands to gain by increasing his muscular strength, is frequently an impossible task; after all, he feels he is already superior...so of what use to him is more muscular bulk.

He will probably be superior to many other men with far greater muscular bulk...and since he will almost always fail to understand the actual factors that make him superior, he will probably make the mistake of assuming that increased muscular bulk might actually reduce his performance.

And it is a common mistake, almost a universal mistake...but a terrible mistake; a mistake that literally prevents the best athletes from reaching their real potential. The very men who stand to gain the most from strength training are usually afraid to try it. Fifty years from now, all athletes in all sports will use strength training as one of the most important parts of their training...at which time they probably still will not understand why it is of such great importance; but they will, at least, believe in strength train-

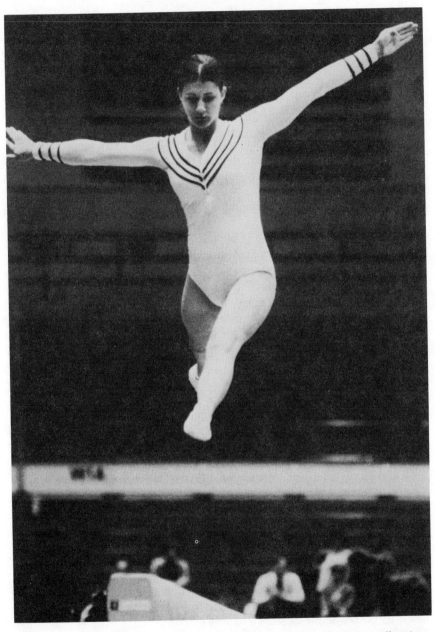

When and if the next great leap forward comes in sports, it will be a direct result of proper strength training...but it will occur only when the present attitude of fear is gone, only when the old myths and superstitions have died, if they ever do.

ing...and they will have lost their fear of strength training.

In the meantime, millions of athletes and thousands of coaches are almost desperately looking for some sort of an edge, literally anything to give them an advantage; while continuing to ignore the one remaining edge, the one factor that is seldom exploited, strength training.

Strength training will not make a superman out of an average man, and nothing else will either. But it will improve the performance of any athlete in any sport.

And it will not make him slower...in fact, it will make him faster.

And it will not reduce his flexibility...in fact, it will increase his flexibility.

And while it will do absolutely nothing to help his skill...it will do nothing to hurt it either.

And it will not make him immune to injury...but it will greatly reduce his chances of injury.

The muscles are the engine of the body; the muscles produce force...the muscles produce movement...the muscles provide energy. Without muscles a person would be utterly helpless, unable to move; yet, here we are in the last quarter of the twentieth century and most coaches and athletes are still literally afraid of their muscles.

When (and if) the next great leap forward comes in sports, it will be a direct result of proper strength training but it will occur only when the present attitude of fear is gone, only when the old myths and superstitions have died, if they ever do.

In the meantime, in many ways, the situation is getting worse instead of better...primarily because a whole new set of myths and superstitions are currently being added to the old ones; many of these false beliefs are concerned with the human nervous system and its relationship to functional ability.

The nervous system itself is not capable of improvement...but a person can, and he certainly should, improve his ability to make use of the system that he does have. The development of skill is nothing more or less than an improvement in the use of the nervous system; but the potential for improving the use of the nervous system does not stop with the development of skill.

Instinct plays a far more important role in human activities than most people realize, or like to admit, even when they do suspect its importance...and instinct, even though it produces automatic reactions more or less beyond our control, can still be used to great advantage. The stretch reflex is a good example of such a usable instinct.

Muscles are arranged in pairs...one set of muscles on one side of a joint for the purpose of bending at that joint, and another set of muscles on the opposite side of the same joint for the purpose of straightening the arm at the joint of the elbow.

The Nervous System in Sports

The muscles in front of the elbow joint, primarily the biceps, bend the arm...the muscles in the rear of the elbow, the triceps, straighten the arm. Similar situations exist on both sides of all human joints, although many are far more complex than the muscles involved in movement around the elbow joint.

Depending upon the desired direction of movement at the moment, these opposite working sets of muscles are called either agonist muscles or antagonist muscles...an agonist muscle produces movement by contraction...while an antagonist muscle limits or stops movement by refusing to permit itself to be stretched.

In order for movement to occur, an agonist muscle must reduce its length, contract with a pulling force that produces movement...but simultaneously, the antagonist muscle must permit movement, by allowing its length to be increased. Thus, during all movements, while one set of muscles is getting shorter, another set of muscles must be getting longer.

It is obvious, then, that a person must relax the muscles on one side of a joint in order to produce movement by contracting the muscles on the other side of the same joint; and in practice, he does this automatically, instinctively, and probably without even being aware that he is doing so.

In any activity involving sudden movement, a person must relax the antagonist muscles instinctively because it occurs so rapidly that there simply is not enough time for thought. So the nervous system provides this service on an instinctive level, as it must.

But...even though this occurs instinctively and automatically, it does not follow that we must remain unaware of this instinct; nor does it follow that we cannot control this instinct to some degree, thus using it for our own purposes.

In fact, very valuable use of the stretch reflex can be made in proper strength training...and should be, but with knowledge and an understanding of the involved factor, so the use of this instinct will produce good results instead of injuries. Using this instinct properly will lead to an increase in the results produced by strength training...using it improperly will almost certainly produce injury.

The stretch reflex is one of several protective instincts of the body. It is intended to keep a person from hurting himself. When sudden movements occur anywhere in the body, the antagonist muscles almost instantly come into play to stop that movement...because, if rapid movement is allowed to continue to the end of the possible range of movement, then damage will probably be done to either the muscular structures or the joints.

A person's arm can straighten only so far, and if it reaches that limit while moving at a high rate of speed then something will be damaged; so the stretch reflex comes into play, sends a signal through the nervous system to trigger the action of the antagonist muscles, and either slows or stops the movement, thus reducing the chance of injury.

All of this is well and good...but it does not stop here. The same stretch reflex is used by our bodies for an entirely different purpose...as an aid to functional ability, and as a means of increasing our usable strength, making it possible for us to jump higher, hit harder, and throw a greater distance.

When a person punches with his fist, he draws his arm back first...but not for the reason that he probably thinks; he does not draw back his fist immediately prior to a punch in order to give the fist a greater range of movement. Instead, he does so in order to bring the stretch reflex into play...the result being that he literally has two separate sets of muscle fibers working for him at the same time when he punches. He has one set of muscle fibers that are working normally, under his control, and another set of fibers that are working instinctively as a result of the stretch reflex.

When a person suddenly pulls back his arm before a punch, he automatically triggers the stretch reflex, which then brings the antagonist muscles into play to stop the sudden movement to the rear. Then, while these fibers are working to slow or stop the rearward movement, he reverses the action and contracts the punching muscle. These muscles are already working as a result of the stretch reflex. The result is that much higher than normal percentages of the muscles become involved in the punch, the punch travels faster, and he hits harder.

Exactly the same thing occurs when a person dips just before jumping or when he backswings with a baseball bat. A similar utilization of pre-stretch inadvertently occurs in golf, tennis, bowling, and most other active sports.

If a person stopped a barbell at the bottom and then started from a stationary position, he might be able to bench press 300 pounds...but if, instead, he allowed the barbell to drop slightly just before starting to press, then he might be able to bench press 350 pounds, or more.

And...I certainly am not suggesting that a person bounce the barbell off his chest; bouncing has absolutely nothing to do with it. The increased usable strength is a result of the stretch reflex. The same thing can easily be demonstrated even when the barbell never touches the chest. For example, take a weight that is slightly below maximum for one repetition, stop the movement with the barbell about an inch above the chest, and then start the first repetition from a dead stop...then, during the second repetition, stop the barbell again when it is an inch above the chest, and then start the first repetition from a dead stop...then, during the second repetition, stop the barbell when it is an inch above the chest; but this time do not start from that position...instead, let the barbell drop a distance of only half an inch, still do not touch the chest, and instantly start to press. A person will find that the second repetition is actually easier than the first one, even though he will obviously be weaker by that point in the exercise. The second repetition will be easier because of the help he is getting as a result of the stretch reflex.

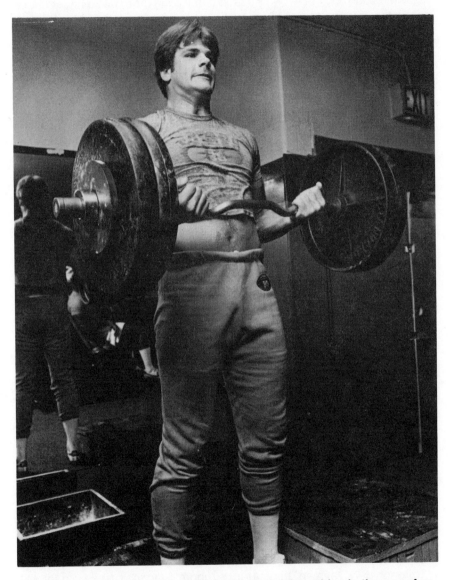

The practice of fast lifts will build little or absolutely nothing in the way of actual strength in the muscles...instead, a person will learn the skill required to throw a barbell; that is right, throw a barbell...because he certainly is not lifting it.

So far, so good...but do not make the dangerous mistake of going too far in this direction. Do not wrongly assume that a big drop will be better than a small drop; it will not be. A very short, very brief drop is all that is required, and a longer drop may well produce an opposite result, thus making a person weaker. And a longer drop will certainly produce a dangerous situation that can easily cause injury.

Triggering of the stretch reflex occurs in microseconds, literally in a tiny fraction of a second. It takes very little to set this instinct to work; more is certainly not better in this instance.

On the contrary, prolonged stretching will actually reduce a person's momentary strength.

And, of equal importance, a longer drop of the weight will build up a high level of momentum in the barbell; force will be trying to move in the opposite direction...an additional force that a person will be required to overcome in order to press the weight. Even the slight, short drop of a properly executed repetition will add some force in the wrong direction, but the extra reflex will more than compensate.

At the moment, an enormous amount of controversy exists on the subject of speed of movement during strength training exercises; so, I feel that it is of great importance that what I am saying here is not misunderstood. I am not suggesting sudden movement, I am not recommending a so-called explosive style of training; on the contrary, the facts are perfectly clear on this point at least...sudden or jerky movements should be avoided during strength training exercises. They have absolutely nothing to offer except the danger of injury.

The movement that occurs during an explosive lift literally occurs so fast that the muscles are unable to keep up...the result being that the involved muscles are exposed to a dangerous jerk at the start of the movement, and then are not involved at all during most of the movement,.

The practice of fast lifts will build little or absolutely nothing in the way of actual strength in the muscles, instead, a person will learn the skill required to throw a barbell; that is right, throw a barbell...because he certainly is not lifting it.

For a weight lifter such skills are a necessary thing...but they are utterly useless for any other athlete; and developing the skill to throw a barbell is unavoidably dangerous, a danger to which active athletes should never be exposed.

Unfortunately, many of the current strength coaches come from the old school, being former weight lifters themselves. As weight lifters, they had to train in that manner in order to develop the skills required for weight lifting; so it naturally follows that they pass on this style of training to other athletes, football players in particular.

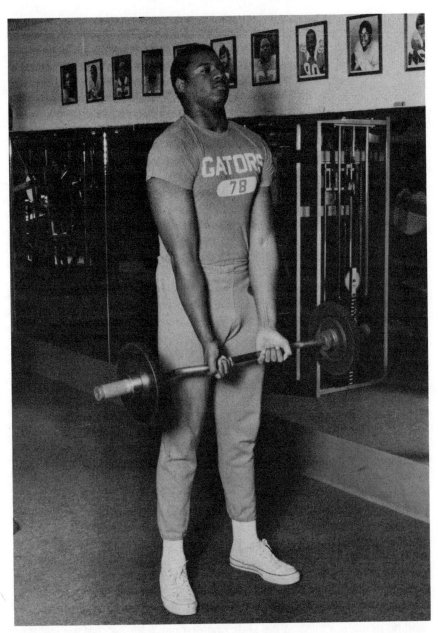

The barbell can be, and properly used will be, a valuable tool for a football player or almost any other athlete, in any sport...but the barbell should be used for the purpose of increasing strength, not for the dangerous and useless purpose of developing skill at throwing a barbell.

The result is that many thousands of football players and other athletes are now being forced to take part in a style of training that is of absolutely no value for the purpose of developing actual muscular strength...and far worse, a style of training that is extremely dangerous. The so-called power clean is one common example of a lift that is of no value to anybody except a weight lifter, and is a very dangerous lift to practice.

So I am against weight lifting, right? Wrong. I have lifted weights for more than thirty-five years; for a long time in an explosive fashion, until I learned better...the hard way.

I am not against hitting and blocking either for a football player...because this is absolutely the only way that a football player will ever learn to hit and block. But it would be outright insanity to suggest that a swimmer or a basketball player should also practice hitting and blocking.

And it is equally insane to suggest that football players should engage in activities that are required for a weight lifter...but are of no value to a football player. Yet this is exactly what is happening in literally thousands of cases, simply from a lack of knowledge.

The barbell can be, and if properly used will be, a valuable tool for a football player, or almost any other athlete in any sport, but the barbell should be used for the purpose of increasing strength, not for the dangerous and useless purpose of developing skill at throwing a barbell.

During the course of the last three years, I have been both directly and indirectly involved in an activity that I have never before mentioned in print, even though, during these same three years I have published more than two dozen articles on strength training in several periodicals. I have avoided any mention of this activity for what I consider to be a very good reason...because I was afraid it would be misunderstood, and might lead to bad results rather than good results.

But now I will take what I consider to be the calculated risk of mentioning this subject in print...hoping that it will be understood and applied in context, but rather expecting that it will not be.

In the state of Florida, where I live, weight lifting is a high school sport. But, like all other sports, it is not practiced at every high school in the state; thus, until three years ago, weightlifting was not one of the sports practiced or engaged in by the DeLand High School. But for three years, it has been.

And...for three years, starting from scratch with no previous training or experience, the weight lifting team of the DeLand School has won every single meet it has entered. As of this moment, their record is 34 wins, no ties, and no defeats, including the state championship for each of the last three years.

The DeLand weight lifters train with barbells and with *Nautilus* equipment, and a large and important part of their training consists of negative-only exercises...where the weight is lowered slowly, but is never lifted.

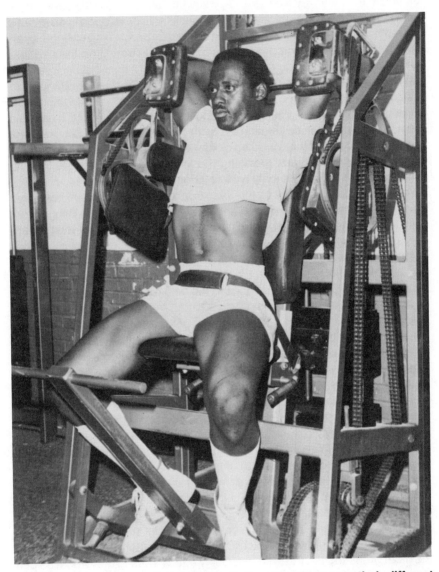

Building strength is one thing...demonstrating strength is an entirely different matter.

The skill required to lift a barbell explosively, to throw a barbell, is developed in the only way it can be...by throwing barbells; but the strength required to produce a truly outstanding weight lifter is developed in an entirely different manner, also in the only way it can be, by performing strength exercises with smooth, slow movement, and by concentrating on the negative parts of all movements.

My personal involvement with the DeLand High School weight lifting team has consisted of providing the required training equipment, including most of the barbells even though I do not manufacture or sell barbells. It has also consisted of a very close relationship with the team's coach, Bill Bradford. Coach Bradford and I have worked closely together on a number of projects over a period of six years, including the long-range experiments that we conducted with a negative-only type of training.

We do not claim to know all the answers...but we do at least know what works best; now we are trying to find out exactly why certain things work best...hoping that such knowledge can then be put to use in a practical manner that will produce even better results.

And we also know some things that do not work at all, or very poorly...things that are dangerous, things that should be avoided. Heading the list of useless, dangerous things in the field of strength training is a so-called explosive style of training, lifts such as the power clean, clean and jerk, and snatch.

We also know that very brief but hard training is actually far more than a possibility...in fact, it is an outright requirement for good results from strength training. During the West Point study, for example, we produced an average increase in neck strength of nearly 92 percent in a group of 18 football players in a period of only six weeks, as a result of only 12 workouts of approximately 8 minutes each.

Two brief weekly workouts, for a period of only six weeks...a training time of approximately 90 minutes, produced approximately a 1 percent increase in neck strength from each minute of training.

Fine and good, but perhaps even more training would have produced a better result. But, in fact, it appears that more training will actually reduce the production of results. Two other groups of West Point cadets trained for a shorter period of time, only four weeks and without supervision; one group trained twice weekly and increased their strength about 42 percent...while the other group trained three times weekly and increased only about 39 percent. So, on the basis of this study, it appears that three weekly workouts actually produce less results than two weekly workouts...and if this is true, then just what is the point of the extra weekly workout?

We intend to find out, in the only way possible, by conducting a long-range research program with a large number of subjects. But research alone is not enough. It must be carefully supervised research. Every single repetition of every exercise in every workout must be performed and recorded under close supervision. If not, then we can never be quite certain just what actually was done, and what was not done.

And it must be done right out in the open, where anybody can watch and the pre-experiment and post-experiment testing must be done by outside experts, by people who are in no way involved in the experiment except for testing purposes. And there must be non-trained control groups who are also tested, and all testing must be done on a blind basis where the testers do not know whether a subject is a member of an experimental group or a control group.

So research can be, and should be, a very valuable course of valid and useful information, but only when it is conducted properly...which, in the real world, it seldom is.

It seldom is simply because most people who undertake research do not have the financial resources, the time, or the facilities required to do it properly. And, secondly, properly conducted research becomes very boring in short order; so it also requires a staff that is highly motivated, people who will devote the time and close attention that are absolutely essential to meaningful results.

Handing a project over to a graduate student and turning your back will not hack it; but in practice, this is what usually happens. Try coaching a football team in the same manner and see how long a coach keeps his job.

Up to this point in time, my company, *Nautilus Sports/Medical Industries*, has been a non-profit organization...simply because every cent that might have been profit has gone directly into research and development, in efforts to improve both the tools available for proper strength training and the use of these tools.

This situation will continue for at least several more years until we reach a point where it is literally impossible to devote the additional resources to meaningful research.

In the last six years alone we have introduced a number of valuable innovations into strength training...1) full-range exercise...2) rotary-form exercise...3) stretching...4) pre-stretching...5) direct resistance...6) variable resistance...7) balanced resistance...8) omnidirectional resistance...9) resistance in a position of muscular contraction...10) negative-only exercise...11) negative-accentuated exercise...12) hyper-exercise...13) infirmetric exercise...14) brief but hard exercise...and a number of other important factors. Every one of these factors is a direct result of our long-range and continuing research programs; and the value of all of these factors has been proven and proven again by careful research.

The type of training that we are now recommending may not be the ultimate; improvements are almost certain to come in the future...but it is, at least, so far ahead of whatever type is in second place that no meaningful comparison is even possible.

And it should be clearly understood that the style of training we are recommending is usable with almost any type of equipment...with barbells, with conventional exercise machines, or with *Nautilus* equipment.

Better results will be produced with *Nautilus* equipment for the simple reason that only *Nautilus* equipment provides full-range exercise; but good results can be produced with almost any type of equipment if it is used properly...which it seldom is.

Strength training exercises, practiced in an explosive fashion, will not give athletes explosive power to use on a football field or a basketball court...instead, it will eventually give a high percentage of injuries to their muscles and joints.

Building strength is one thing. Demonstrating strength is an entirely different matter. Do not confuse the two.

16
The Relationship of Strength to Functional Ability in Sports

By Arthur Jones

Functional ability in sports is a product of five factors...but only one of these factors is actually productive. The other four factors are certainly important, but they are not productive...instead, they are supportive in nature.

Skill is simply the ability to make effective use of the force produced by the muscles. But no amount of skill will produce movement...only the muscles produce movement.

Favorable bodily proportions provide an athlete with an enormous advantage. But this advantage is of no value without the strength of his muscles.

Cardiovascular ability is also important...but only in the sense that it permits work; no amount of cardiovascular ability will perform work. Only the muscles perform work.

Neurological efficiency is another factor of great importance...but again, only in the sense that it provides an athlete's muscles with an advantage and permits him to use a higher than average percentage of whatever muscles he has. But, in the end, it is the muscles that produce movement...the muscles that perform work...the muscles that provide energy...and, to a great degree, the muscles that protect an athlete from injury.

Yet...in the face of the previously mentioned simple facts, here we are in the last quarter of the twentieth century, and most people still believe the same old myths that existed centuries ago. In plain English, many coaches and many thousands of athletes are literally afraid of muscles...still fearing that building their muscles will somehow hurt their ability, slow them down, reduce their flexibility, or otherwise limit their performance.

No amount of muscle will help an athlete much if he lacks the skill to use it effectively...but no amount of muscle will hurt his skill either; instead, increasing his strength will always improve his functional ability, in any sport.

An athlete's muscles can be as strong as those of an elephant...but if his bodily proportions are bad for a particular sport, then he still will not be able to perform well. But he will, at least, perform better than he would have with weaker muscles.

A sprinter can have muscles like those of Hercules and still fall flat on his face after a 100-yard dash if his cardiovascular condition is bad...but he should not make the common mistake of assuming that he can have only one or the other, either great strength or good cardiovascular condition but not both. In fact, it is easily possible (and highly desirable) to have both.

One of the most outstanding muscular freaks that I ever saw was actually a fairly weak man...stronger than an average man, but certainly not as strong as one might guess from the size of his muscles. But his lack of strength is in no way related to the size of his muscles; as it happens, this particular individual is very low on the scale of neurological ability; he lacks the ability to utilize a large part of his actual muscular mass...a genetic problem that is not subject to improvement.

But even this man, weak as he is, is still far more capable than he would have been with smaller, weaker muscles.

Given this man's muscular size, plus favorable bodily proportions, great skill, outstanding neurological ability, and good cardiovascular condition...the result would be almost literally a superman. One day we will see such a specimen...and then, when the actual possibilities become evident to a large number of people, we will soon thereafter see quite a lot of such men.

If Dick Butkus had ever bothered to train his muscles (and he never did until it was too late to do him much good)...we would be looking at such a superman right now. Dick was probably the best in the world at his particular specialty...but not as a result of great strength; instead, he was a naturally strong man who also happened to have every possible advantage for a particular activity...great skill, ideal bodily proportions for a specific function, at least adequate cardiovascular ability for the same function, and outstanding neurological efficiency. Given these advantages he was the best in the world with absolutely nothing in the way of strength training. This might lead many people to believe that he did not need strength training, that it might even have hurt him in some fashion...when, in fact, Dick had far more to gain from such training than most have. He now realizes this after the fact, too late to be of any help.

This is certainly not meant to be an indictment of Dick Butkus, he was merely chosen as an example...any one of several hundred other such examples could have been used; and most people would recognize the names of all of them. As it happens, Dick is a close personal friend of mine and a business associate; but that does not change the fact that he utterly

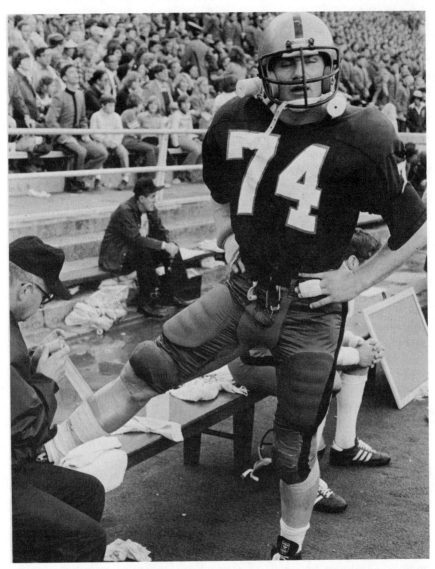

One well-known sports doctor plainly states that 50 percent of all sports-connected injuries could be prevented by proper strength training; which is his opinion, an opinion that I can neither confirm nor deny...but it is certainly obvious that at least some injuries would be prevented, and since there were approximately 300,000 sports injuries last year that required surgical attention, then a reduction of even 10 percent would be an enormous step in the right direction.

failed to realize the value of strength training during most of the nineteen years that he played football, from junior high school through his years with the pros. In this regard he was typical; like most outstanding athletes, he was a natural...a man who appeared to have everything. But who, in fact, was overlooking one of great importance; a factor that could have made him even better than he was—strength training...a factor that would have markedly improved his functional ability, while reducing chances of injury.

Dick, like thousands of other athletes, failed to realize the importance of strength training because nobody ever bothered to tell him about it...while a number of people did tell him all of the old myths, false beliefs, and outright lies that have helped to keep sports away from the actually great value of strength training until very recently.

But now all of that has changed, right? Now everybody understands the value of strength training, right? Wrong...dead wrong. Relatively few people have finally permitted themselves to be convinced, although hesitantly and even fearfully, that there might be some value to strength training in a few cases in some sports. While the vast majority of people connected with sports in any capacity remain almost literally scared to death of strength training, they are still convinced that increasing the strength of an athlete will somehow hurt his performance.

In the meantime, it has been clearly and repeatedly demonstrated hundreds of times, with no single exception I ever heard of and no exception I would believe unless I saw it myself, that proper strength training will markedly improve the performance of any athlete in any sport.

And the great athletes are the ones who have the most to gain from strength training...and are the most unlikely to use it; having been falsely convinced that it will hurt them.

Proper strength training may improve the functional ability of a clod by as much as 50 percent...but he will still be a clod, and will still be run over by untrained athletes who have all of the natural advantages that the clod lacks. But even a 2 percent improvement in the functional ability of a natural athlete may well be the difference between a good athlete and a world champion.

And just how much improvement can be produced by proper strength training? An impossible question, obviously. It depends upon the particular activity involved, the individual involved, and many other factors. But...in all cases, in all sports, there will be a measurable degree of improvement; to a level of performance that would never have been reached by that individual without proper strength training.

And what degree of protection against injury will be provided by proper strength training? Another impossible question, since too many factors are again involved. But it should be obvious that a strong limb is far less likely to be injured than a weak one is, and it is well established that strength training increases not only the size and strength of the muscles, but the connective tissues and even the bones.

One well-known sports doctor plainly states that 50 percent of all sports-connected injuries could be prevented by proper strength training; which is his opinion, an opinion that I can neither confirm nor deny...but it is certainly obvious that at least some injuries would be prevented, and since there were approximately 300,000 sports injuries last year that required surgical attention, then a reduction of even 10 percent would be an enormous step in the right direction.

The proper tool for that giant step is in existence right now, and is being used by thousands of people...while being ignored by millions of other people. Proper strength training is the tool. Use it. An athlete has everything to gain, and nothing to lose except problems and while it certainly will not solve all of his problems, would it not be wise for him to settle for a solution to some of his problems?

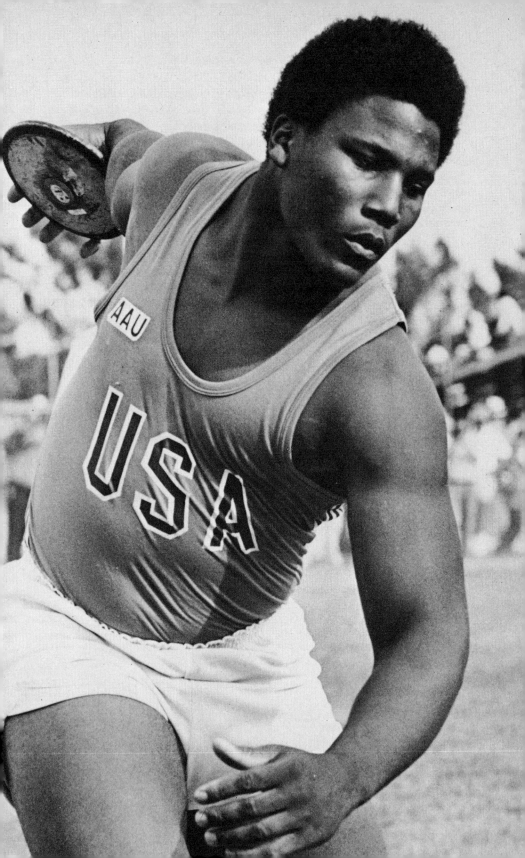

17
Specificity in Strength Training - The Facts and Fables

By Arthur Jones

Do not be misled...and you can be, on the subject of specificity.

There are no degrees of specificity...either you have it, or you do not. A movement is either utterly specific, or it is not specific at all.

This being true, as it is, it obviously follows that the only possible way to produce specificity in anything is by performing the act itself. In effect, the only possible specific training for basketball is the act of playing basketball...the only possible specific training for swimming is swimming itself, and so on.

Strength is general, and contributes to any activity...but the applied demonstration of strength is specific. Learning to apply your strength properly in any activity requires skill training...not strength training, but skill training and skill training can come from only one possible source, the practice of the sport itself.

If it were possible, which it is not, to design an exercise in such a way that it was nearly specific, then the use of such an exercise would hurt you far more than it could help you. And the closer it came to being specific, the worse it would hurt you.

All intelligent coaches are clearly aware that practice carried beyond a certain point is of no value...that it may actually produce a reduction in skill. Why? Simply because a tired athlete changes his style of performance. He begins performing his movements differently, as he must to compensate for his reduced strength, the unavoidable result being that he learns two or more different styles of performance...a fresh style and a tired style, so to speak.

He forms two or more sets of motor memories, which inevitably leads to confusion...and his performances suffer as a result.

One of the oldest tricks in the world of sport, if bullfighting can be called a sport, is directly related to specificity. The night before a bull is to be fought, his horns are shortened by approximately a quarter of an inch...the next day, before he has become accustomed to his shorter horns, he goes into the ring to fight and die.

And there stands the brave matador, being barely missed by the enraged bull...being missed by one-quarter of an inch, being missed by the amount that the bull's horns were shortened.

The bull knows exactly where the tips of his horns are, if he must use them effectively. Shortening his horns by as little as a quarter of an inch will cause him to miss his target entirely.

Did you ever get a grain of sand inside of your sock? It feels like a boulder and changes your entire style of walking or running...then, when you finally get it out, it turns out to be so small that you can barely see it.

True specificity is just that exact, and hitting or missing the target can easily be determined by far less than a quarter of an inch or a grain of sand.

While I am clearly aware in advance that the following example will undoubtedly infuriate at least some of my readers; nevertheless it illustrates my present point rather clearly...so I will use it.

I have been a hunter for nearly 50 years, for sport, as a business, and in connection with wildlife conservation work...in this country, in South America, in India, in Australia, in Malaya, but mainly in Africa. During these years I have hunted just about everything that walks, crawls, swims or flies, from quail to elephant, including men.

I hunted for quail for sport and for food, killing them...most of the other animals were captured alive, for translocation to animal parks or for relocation in areas of safety...but in some cases I have killed animals in connection with wildlife conservation work; such controlled hunting is called just that, control hunting...a carefully calculated thinning out of the herds when an overpopulation of animals reaches a point where the habitat itself is being damaged.

A given area of land can contain and feed a limited number of animals, and when the number of animals passes a certain point, then the habitat itself will be destroyed and all of the animals will die. So herds have to be thinned out, numbers have to be reduced...to save many animals, some animals must die. Some years ago in Africa, this was my job...and during that stage of my career, I personally killed more than 600 elephants, which, in that business, is actually rather small. When I moved back to this country from Africa, nine years ago, several men that I knew personally were killing at least 1,000 elephants a year, 1,000 each, every year for a period of many years.

This is certainly not sport and it is certainly not fun...it is, instead, outright butchery; even if, as happens to be the case, necessary butchery.

There is no stalking of lone tuskers, little or no danger to the hunters, no romance, no adventure...instead, you pick out a particular herd and then kill the entire herd, bulls, cows, juveniles and even babies. Remember, the idea is to reduce the number of elephants within a particular area; and this must be done by killing elephants of both sexes and all sizes in order to preserve a balance of sexes and sizes.

So you select a herd of 40 or 50 elephants, or more...and then, in something under three minutes you kill them all. When the shooting is over, the bodies are literally stacked up.

To a witness of such a slaughter, things happen so fast that the result is nothing short of outright shock...one moment a herd of elephants is moving slowly by, and the next moment they are all dead. The shots come so thick and fast, and the elephants drop so suddenly and in such numbers, that a man seeing this for the first time literally cannot believe his own eyes.

Two men who know what they are doing can kill an entire herd of 50 elephants in less than a minute...each man will drop an elephant approximately every two seconds...one shot, one elephant. And it must be done in this fashion...because, if the herd has time to realize what is happening, some will escape. Then, the next time they run across a man, perhaps a poor unarmed African on a bicycle...well, look out, elephants have long memories. So you must kill the entire herd and leave no survivors anxious to even the score.

I have been personally involved in such slaughters, on the shooting end, at least 30 times, and have been a non-shooting witness to another 50 or so slaughters...none of which experiences give me any prideful memories, but all of which actions were utterly necessary, even if unpleasant.

In such a situation, when the action starts, there is literally no time for thought...instead of thinking, you react, instinctively, in accord with your learned and practiced skills.

Afterwards, a first-time witness to such a slaughter will invariably ask you a certain question...a question I have been asked many times, and a question that I could not even begin to answer until recently.

"Where do you aim," they ask, "in order to hit the brain?"

I never could answer that question because the aiming point is always different...if a big elephant is close, with his head high, then you might shoot in the mouth...turned away, you might shoot behind the ear...facing you at an angle, in front of the ear...but never in the same place twice.

But I could never tell someone else where to aim...because, you see, I was not shooting at the elephant at all; instead, I was shooting at the elephant's brain...and since it made no difference what part of the elephant was between my gun and his brain, I did not even notice the external part of the elephant where I aimed.

I knew where the elephant's brain was located. I aimed at the brain, and the fact that my bullet had to pass through some other part of the elephant in order to reach the brain was utterly irrelevant.

And...you do exactly the same thing in any sporting activity; you do not think about it, you simply do it...there is literally no time for thought, so your reflexes have to be exactly right, exactly right.

For elephants I used a double-barreled .600 caliber rifle as long as I could get ammunition for it...then, I was forced to change guns due to a lack of ammunition for my old standby. I could not hit a thing at first; not while shooting as fast as possible, at least.

Why? Because my reflexes were attuned to an exact skill, with a certain tool...total specificity. The newer tool was supposed to be better, and it might have been more accurate from a bench rest position, but I certainly could not use it accurately while shooting quickly.

The point should now be perfectly clear...there is only one possible way to obtain specificity, by performing the act itself, with the same tool, in exactly the same manner.

An exercise that is nearly specific will simply mess up your skills...an exercise that is almost specific will have the same bad result. So do not try to be specific in your exercises...in any case, doing so is impossible, and the closer you come, the greater the danger of hurting your skill.

Build strength in the best way possible...with little or absolutely no regard to how that strength is to be used; then learn to use that strength to your greatest advantage in the only way possible, by practice of the sport itself.

Adding a few ounces to the weight of a basketball will do absolutely nothing in the way of increasing your strength for playing basketball...but it certainly will ruin your skill in basketball.

Adding a few pounds to the weight of a basketball will do very little in the way of increasing your strength...and it will still have some bad effect on your skill, although not as much as the previous example.

So it is obvious that the closer we come to having specificity, the worse off we are...until and unless we have total specificity, in which case we are simply throwing a normal basketball in our usual fashion, which will increase our skill while doing nothing for our strength.

Build the muscles that are involved in basketball, or any sport...and build them the best and fastest way you can; without trying to be specific, without trying to duplicate the action of the sport itself.

Anything else is insanity. Anything else will hurt you far more than it helps you.

I fly my own airplanes an average of nearly 1,000 hours a year, and I have now flown a total in excess of 23,000 hours over a period of nearly 38 years. I am still the holder of a current airline transport license...yet, this very day,

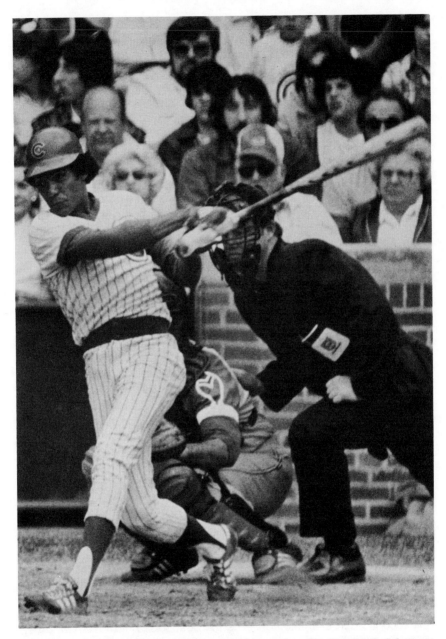

Strength is general, and contributes to any activity...but the applied demonstration of strength is specific; and learning to apply your strength properly in any activity requires skill training...not strength training, but skill training can come from only one possible source, the practice of the sport itself.

when I flew a Cherokee 6 for the first time in about three months, I could instantly tell that my skill in that airplane was far below par.

I have owned three airplanes exactly like that one during the last twelve years and have a total of at least 3,000 hours of experience in such planes, but it still did not feel quite right to me after less than three months out of practice...even though I have flown other airplanes approximately 200 hours during that period of three months.

To build your skills...or even to retain your skills...you must practice any activity with total specificity. For the last three months I have been flying a jet only, and when I went back to the Cherokee 6, my reflexes were wrong...not wrong enough to get me killed, not wrong enough to keep me from flying the airplane safely, but certainly wrong enough to keep me from doing a perfect job of flying, wrong enough to make the difference between winning or losing any sort of contest of flying skill against an equally qualified pilot who has been flying the Cherokee regularly.

So flying the jet did not help me in flying the Cherokee...in fact, it hurt me, because it was slightly different...not greatly different, just slightly different. If the difference had really been great, then the jet experience would not have hurt my skill.

Years ago, I used to fly a heavy bomber and an earlier model Cherokee...and the experience in one did not hurt my skill in the other, because the difference was great.

I could belabor the point into the ground, and perhaps I already have...but I am concerned when I read claims being made that are apparently based on outright insanity, dangerously false claims, grossly misleading claims.

At this point in time (March 6, 1977), the entire field of strength training is up to its ears in myth, superstition, fear, doubt, ignorance, and outright lies...and while I make no claims that I know all of the answers, at least a few simple facts are perfectly clear.

Specificity in strength training is an outright myth, an utter impossibility...and it is a good thing it is impossible, because it has absolutely no value in the way of increasing strength; and...anything approaching specificity is even worse, because it will do little or nothing to increase strength but it will hurt your skills.

Some of the same people who have been doing so much talking recently about the supposed advantages of specificity in strength training are also responsible for the spreading of other fables of equal value...in other words, no value.

A second such example concerns the best speed of movement during exercise. A third example concerns the supposed differences between the so-called fast-twitch and slow-twitch muscle fibers.

You must move suddenly, they say...fast exercise produces fast muscles, they claim. Hogwash...pure unadulterated garbage, utterly false and

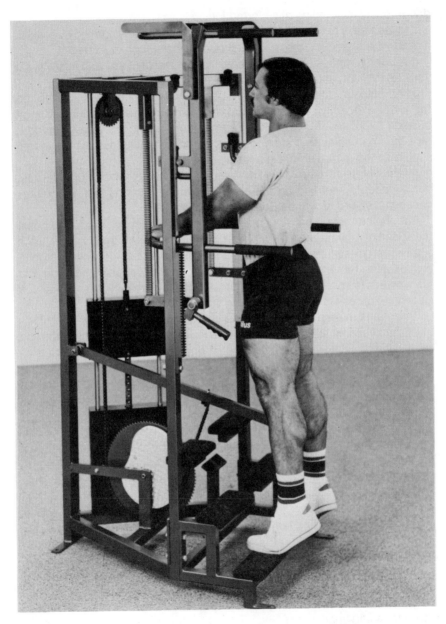

Build strength in the best way possible...with little or absolutely no regard to how that strength is to be used; then learn to use that strength to your greatest advantage in the only way possible, by practice of the sport itself.

dangerously misleading misinformation.

It takes heavy resistance to build strength...absolutely nothing else will do it. And...the faster you move, the lighter the resistance must be.

It is utterly impossible to lift a heavy weight rapidly...you can throw it, but you cannot lift it; and throwing weight will not build strength.

In an obvious attempt to mislead people who are not aware of the real facts, it has recently been stated that you must move rapidly during strength building exercises. Move at 136 degrees per second, they say, hoping to give the impression that such a speed of movement is fast...when, in fact, such a speed of movement is actually quite slow.

A fast athlete can move his limbs at a speed in excess of 2,000 degrees per second...something on the order of twenty times as fast as their so-called fast speed of 136 degrees per second.

But...he cannot do so while moving against resistance. Maximum possible speed of movement is possible only when there is literally no resistance, against zero resistance. Then, if you add even a slight amount of resistance, the resulting movement will be slower. And the more resistance you add, the slower the speed will be...until, at last, when you reach the highest possible level of resistance, the resulting speed will be zero.

When maximum possible speed is being produced, then every slightest bit of the available strength is being used to accelerate the mass of the limb itself...and absolutely no remainder of strength is available to overcome resistance.

Then, if resistance is added, you must reduce the speed of movement...nothing else is even possible, and anyone who claims otherwise is either a fool, a liar or both.

So...since it is obvious that heavy resistance unavoidably requires slow movement, and since it is well established and beyond dispute that heavy resistance is required for building strength...it unfailingly follows that proper strength training literally demands a fairly slow rate of movement.

In the state of Florida, competitive weight lifting is a sport at the high school level...but, until five years ago, the DeLand, Florida, high school had never had a weight lifting team.

But they do now...starting from scratch five years ago, with no previous experience to go on while competing with other schools that did have previous experience. The DeLand high school team has now won 55 meets in a row. Never tied, never defected, state champions during each of the last four years and apparently well on the way to repeating that unbeaten, untied record for a fifth year.

And how do they train? Primarily with pure negative work, performed in a very slow fashion, as slowly as possible. Such training builds raw strength. They then learn to use their strength by practicing the specific lifts involved in their sport; the bench press and the clean and jerk; the bench press being a fairly slow lift and the clean and jerk being a very fast lift.

If the resistance is heavy enough, then it does not matter how slowly you move during strength training exercises. In fact, if the resistance is as heavy as it must be for producing good results, then you will literally be forced to move quite slowly, very slowly.

The third fable being bandied about at the moment concerns the supposed differences between the so-called fast-twitch and slow-twitch muscle fibers. At this point in time, nobody knows anything of the slightest value on this subject.

When and if we are able to determine the facts in this matter, regardless of what facts may be, so long as they really are facts, then we will publish the facts in clear detail. In the meantime, however, if you are interested in fables, then you can read all sorts of stated opinions based on outright distortion, guesswork, and simple lies.

But what does science say? Quite frankly, almost anything you want to hear. The scientific community has largely deteriorated into a pure bureaucracy primarily interested in perpetuating itself; the name of the game being research grants...and, publish or perish, with little or no regard for the value of what is actually being published.

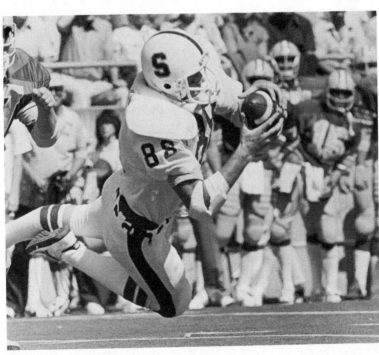

...there is only one possible way to obtain specificity, by performing the act itself, with the same tool, in exactly the same manner.

Specificity in Strength Training - The Facts and Fables

I am all in favor of the stated purpose of science, an unbiased search for truth...unfortunately, as someone recently said, science is contaminated with people. Being people, it unavoidably follows that at least some scientists like money; thus, hardly a day passes that I fail to get at least one letter from some well known scientist offering his services in research in return for my money, of course...and they usually make it quite clear that the results of their research will exactly match my expectations.

In plain English, many scientists will lie for money...and quite a number of them are doing just that at the moment. Well, I need the help of such people as much as I need another hole in my head...so we closely supervise our own research with the cooperation of very carefully checked scientists who do not stand to gain a cent from their work in this field.

I personally do not believe that honest research can be done for money. And right or wrong in that opinion, I will not touch it with a ten foot pole.

So we spend a great deal of money for research, far more than everybody else in this field combined, but that money does not go to pay anyone performing this research. We are interested in the simple truth, whatever it turns out to be, and it just happens that the truth has a way of hiding itself when money becomes involved.

At this very moment we are completing constuction of a 90,000 square foot building, more than two acres under one roof, and this building will contain the largest and best equipped human performance laboratory in the world for the sole purpose of conducting large-scale long range research into every area of physiology related to human performance.

Some people would have you believe that they already know all the answers. Well, I do not claim to know any of the answers, and I am not even too sure about a lot of the questions. If I was, then I would not need to do more research...but since I do not know the answers, we plan a great deal more research, literally as much as we have time and resources for. Perhaps some day we will know a few final answers...but in the meantime, we do at least know what works best at the present state of the art, and we know quite a number of things that do not work at all regardless of the claims made about them.

But even when research is conducted with a total lack of bias, which it seldom is...and even when research is conducted under the best possible conditions, it still follows, unavoidably, that a large part of the conclusions are tainted with subjectivity for the simple reason that the absolute facts are really never known.

Two years ago, in the direction of removing subjectivity (that is to say, opinion) from research, I started work on a totally computerized type of exercise...an exercise device linked to a computer in such a way that the computer would perform two functions; first, the computer will direct the athlete, telling him exactly what to do, how to do it, how fast to do it, how hard

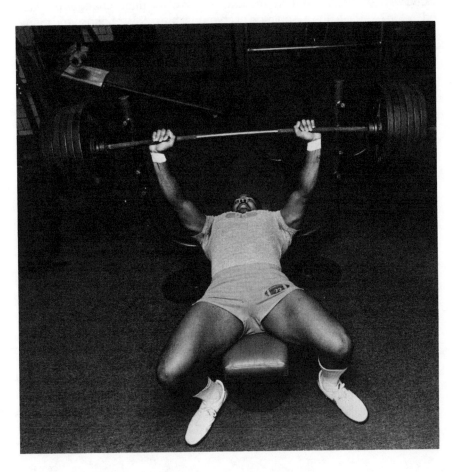

It is utterly impossible to lift a heavy weight rapidly...you can throw it, but you cannot lift it; and throwing weight will not build strength.

to do it, how long to do it...and, secondly, the computer will also make an exact record of what the athlete actually does.

For the first time in the history of strength training, we will be able to determine exactly what has occurred during training...and we will also be provided with an almost perfectly accurate record of the many changes produced by the exercise, the magnitude of changes, the rate of change, and many other important factors that previously involved a great deal of outright guesswork for the simple reason that no accurate method existed for measuring many of the changes produced by exercise.

Within another year at the latest, we will at last be able to conduct research in strength training that is utterly without bias...accurate to a degree almost beyond belief, and then...and only then...will it become possible to determine the final answers to many important questions.

But again...a present lack of final answers does not mean a lack of useful information. On the contrary, we do have a great deal of very practical knowledge. We know a number of things that work very well indeed, producing rapid and steady increases in athletic performances...and, we know a number of things that do not work at all, or work very poorly, and things that are dangerous and should be avoided entirely.

At the moment, in the world of strength training, some people seem to be suffereing from a knee-jerk reflex. If I say up, they say down...if I suggest something is good, they immediately condemn it as being evil...if I say slow, they say fast, and so on. Whatever I say, they immediately say the opposite. Apparently being unable or unwilling to think for themselves, such people merely react...a knee-jerk reflex; I hit a nerve by pointing out the weakness of their previous statements, and they immediately jerk. So I would strongly suggest that you carefully investigate the real facts before attempting to make use of many of the suggestions now being put forth in the world of strength training.

18
Flexibility as a Result
of Exercise

By Arthur Jones

Exercise should increase flexibiity, and it can...but it seldom does. Proper, full-range exercise will increase flexibiity, but improper, mid-range exercise may have an opposite effect.

Contrary to popular opinion, the size of your muscles has absolutely nothing to do with your flexibiity...but the method you use to build those muscles is important. Distance runners normally have very little in the way of muscular size, so you might expect them to be very flexible. In fact, however, quite the opposite is true. As a rule, distance runners have very little flexibility, and many of the injuries so common among distance runners are direct results of their inflexibility.

In contrast, gymnasts are very muscular...and very flexible. So it should be clear that there is no relationship between muscular size and flexibility.

Flexibility is a result of stretching, so exercises that involve stretching will increase flexibilty...while exercises that do not involve stretching will not increase flexibility; such exercises will not, in fact, even prevent a gradual loss of flexibility.

Thus, where possible, exercises should involve stretching...but in practice, very few exercises do involve stretching. In order to provide stretching, the range of movement in an exercise must actually exceed the possible range of movement of the athlete. In effect, you must reach your limit of movement and still encounter resistance. If it is possible to relax in the extended position of an exercise and remove the resistance, then stretching is not provided.

Flexibility as a Result of Exercise

For example, a bench-press does not provide stretching because, at the bottom of the movement, the weight is supported by your chest. In contrast, a properly performed parallel dip exercise provides stretching for the chest and shoulder muscles because in the low position, the resistance is not removed. Regardless of your existing level of flexibility, the resistance will still be imposed even when you have reached the limit of movement. But, please note...I said a properly performed exercise. It is also possible to perform this exercise incorrectly. Unfortunately, this exercise is usually performed incorrectly...and if so, stretching is still not provided.

If the downwards movement is stopped too soon, as it usually is, then the limits of possible movement will never be reached, and stretching will not be provided. So go as low as possible in this exercise...but, a word of warning, do not bounce. Move into the bottom position smoothly and fairly slowly. Do not drop suddenly into this position...dropping into the bottom position of a parallel dip may impose a load of several thousand pounds on your muscles and connective tissues, and might rip them out by the roots.

Performing the exercise properly...that is, going as low as possible and both lifting and lowering the body in a smooth, steady, and fairly slow fashion...will force you to use less resistance; but do not let that disturb you in the least, since an exercise performed incorrectly with a much heavier weight is of little or no value.

You certainly should use as much weight as possible...as much as possible in good form; but do not sacrifice good form for anything. *In exercise, as in most things, good form is frequently the only difference between very good results and no results at all.*

So, for the purpose of increasing flexibility, the choice of exercises is very important, since some exercises provide stretching and some do not...but the style of performance is equally important. In the parallel dip, for example, most people do approximately half the exercise and they do the movements much too fast. Starting at the top, they quickly lower themselves down to about the mid-range of the possible movement, and then they bounce back up to the top as quickly as possible.

By performing the exercise in this manner, you certainly can use more weight, but you certainly will not produce more than a small percentage of the benefits that would have been produced by performing the exercise properly with much less weight.

In one sense, the parallel dip is almost unique. It is one of the few conventional exercises that provides a proper degree of stretching. The only other conventional exercises that provide even a reasonable degree of stretching are the stiff-legged dead lift performed on a bench, the shoulder shrug, the triceps curl performed on an incline bench, the wrist curl performed on a decline bench, heel raises performed on a high block and the full squat.

Again, contrary to popular opinion, most of the exercises that are usually

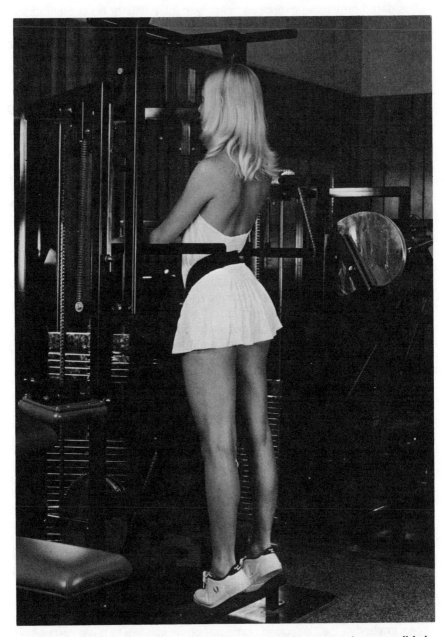

You certainly should use as much weight as possible...as much as possible in good form; but do not sacrifice good form for anything...in exercise, as in most things, good form is frequently the only difference between very good results and no results at all.

considered stretching exercises actually involve little or no stretching. For example, using a wide grip during a pulldown exercise does not provide stretching...on the contrary, a wide grip in this exercise actually reduces the possible range of movement and thus removes the small amount of stretching that might have been done with a much narrower grip.

And the same thing is also true in the bench press. A wide grip does not produce stretching; instead, it actually reduces the amount of stretching provided by a bench press performed with a narrow grip.

A moment's study of illustrations 1 and 2 comparing these two exercises, as performed with both a narrow grip and a wide grip, will make it obvious that in both cases, the wide grip actually reduces the amount of stretching provided. Yet, in practice, most people use a wide grip in these exercises. And if you ask them why, they will usually tell you that a wide grip provides more stretching. And they may believe it...but believing certainly does not make it so.

If we went by what most people believe, then we would never change anything, and without change there could be no improvement. And while I do not mean to imply that change necessarily produces improvement, it should be obvious to anyone that there can be no improvement without change.

And, having changed something, it will then be different, therefore, strange...and most people immediately object to anything the least bit strange because it usually frightens them...frightens them because they do not understand it.

So if you change the style of your exercises, which you should if you have been doing them in the usual fashion, then you can expect some people, perhaps most people, to object.

And their arguments will be many and varied..."Look at the results I produced," some will say. But when they do, then ask yourself just how long it took them...and was it really worth the price?

"Perform the movements as fast as possible," others will say. "Fast movement in exercise builds fast muscles." Hogwash...pure hogwash, very dangerous hogwash, almost criminal hogwash. Fast movements in exercise produce absolutely nothing except injuries.

At this point in time (January, 1977), an enormous controversy exists on the subject of the proper speed of movement during exercise...and this question probably will not be settled to the satisfaction of everybody for many years, if ever.

So...in order to set the record perfectly straight, let it be clearly understood that I do not know the best speed of movement during exercise. But neither does anybody else...although some people would like to have you believe that they do.

But the fact that I do not know the best speed does not mean that I know absolutely nothing on the subject. On the contrary, certain points are obvious. It is obviuos, for example, that a fast speed of movement during exercise is both dangerous and unproductive. Dangerous because it imposes enormous forces on the muscles, connective tissues and joints...and unproductive because it literally removes the resistance from the muscles during a large part of the exercise.

When an exercise movement is performed rapidly, the results are undeniable...first, the forces at the start of the movement are increased enormously, are multiplied by acceleration of the weight...then, secondly, after the weight starts moving, it moves so rapidly that the muscles are literally unable to keep up.

The unavoidable results are that the muscles are yanked very hard at the start of the movement, yanked dangerously hard...and then coast through the rest of the movement against little or no resistance. So such a style of training will produce injuries, but will not produce much if anything in the way of an actual strength increase.

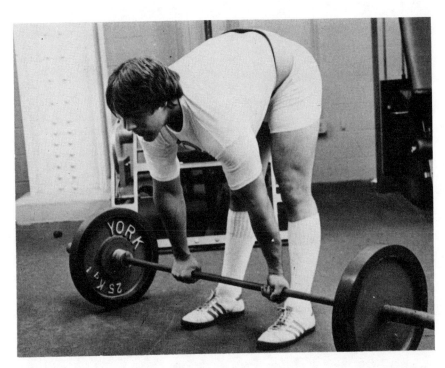

An athlete should not be misled by advice to the effect that he must train explosive strength...such a style of training is the least productive style of training possible, and by far the most dangerous style of training.

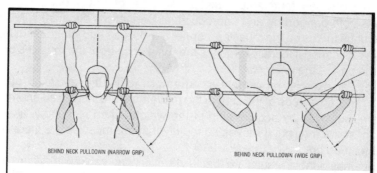

Illustration 1. A wide grip pulldown behind the neck provides a range of movement of 77 degrees, while the same exercise performed with a narrow grip provides approximately 115 degrees of movement...a difference of 38 degrees. If in doubt about which of several exercises to perform, always choose the exercise that involves the greatest range of movement.

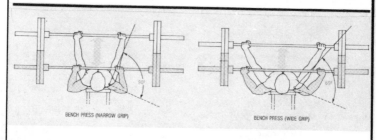

Illustation 2. Notice that the bench press performed with a narrow grip allows approximately 21 degrees more movement than a wide grip style of performance. In neither case, however, does the bench press with a barbell provide much in the way of stretching for the chest and shoulder muscles. A far better conventional exercise for the chest and should muscles is the dipping movement performed between parallel bars.

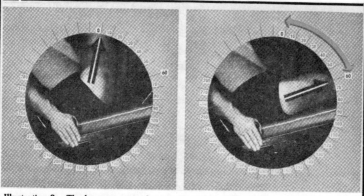

Illustration 3. The leg press provides very limited, mid-range exercise for the hip and thigh muscles. From the starting position to the finishing position, notice that the thigh moves only 60 degrees.

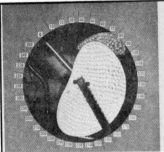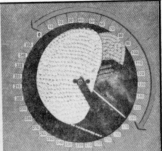

Illustration 4.   In contrast to the leg press, the Nautilus hip and back machine provides a range of movement of the thighs around the hips of over 160 degrees...more than 2½ times that of the leg press. Properly performed repetitions on the hip and back machine will not only increase the flexibility of your athletes, but simultaneously increase their strength throughout a full range of possible movement.

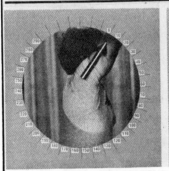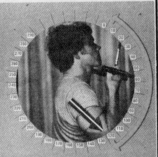

Illustration 5.   Only 120 degrees of movement around the shoulders are provided in the typical pulldown exercise...and there is no resistance in the torso muscles in the starting position or the finishing position.

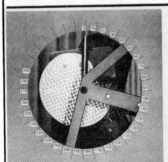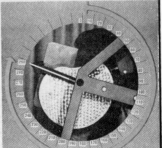

Illustration 6.   Notice that the Nautilus pullover machine provides a possible range of movement around the shoulders of over 280 degrees...an enourmous difference when compared to the pulldown exercise. Furthermore, the pullover machine stretches the torso muscles in the starting position and provides full-range resistance throughout the entire movement, including the position of full muscular contraction.

Yet it probably remains the most commonly used style of training...which also explains why most people produce so very little in the way of worthwhile results, and why training injuries are so common.

So even if the exact answer remains unknown at this time, the question is certainly known...and, properly worded, the question should be, "How slow should we move during exercise? Not how fast...how slow?

And do not be misled into believing that an isokinetic form of exercise provides the answer...it does not. On the contrary, and in spite of many claims, it leaves a great deal to be desired.

Since the subject of this chapter deals primarily with flexibility as a result of exercise, I will restrict my remarks mainly to this area...the area of greatest weakness for any form of isokinetic exercise.

Remember, flexibility is a result of stretching. While it is true that very few conventional exercises provide enough stretching, if any, it is also true that isokinetic exercises provide absolutely no stretching.

Isokinetic resistance is based on friction...which, by its nature, does not provide the back pressure required for stretching. In fact, the makers of isokinetic exercise devices point to this actual fault with apparent pride...hoping, I suppose, to give the impression that a major fault is actually an asset.

Some asset. Without stretching, no exercise of any kind will do anything for flexibiity...and the prolonged practice of exercises that do not provide stretching will actually reduce flexibility.

During the course of an extensive research program conducted at the United States Military Academy, West Point, in April and May of 1975, two groups of varsity football players were compared on the basis of changes in flexibility produced by different styles of training.

Both groups of subjects were involved in spring football practice during the course of the experiment, and both groups were exposed to the normal stretching exercises that form a part of football practice...and both groups were involved in strength training programs, but here there was a difference.

One group was trained exclusively on *Nautilus* equipment...trained very briefly but very hard; a total of only seventeen brief workouts during a period of six weeks...workouts that averaged less than thirty minutes each.

Both groups were carefully tested for flexibility before and after the period of training...and both groups improved their flexibiity as a result of their training, but they did not improve equally.

In the first area of flexibility improvement, the *Nautilus* group improved ten times as much as the conventional group...not 10 percent more, but ten times as much, literally a 1,000 percent increase.

In the second area of improvement, the *Nautilus* group improved eleven times as much as the conventional group, a 1,100 percent increase.

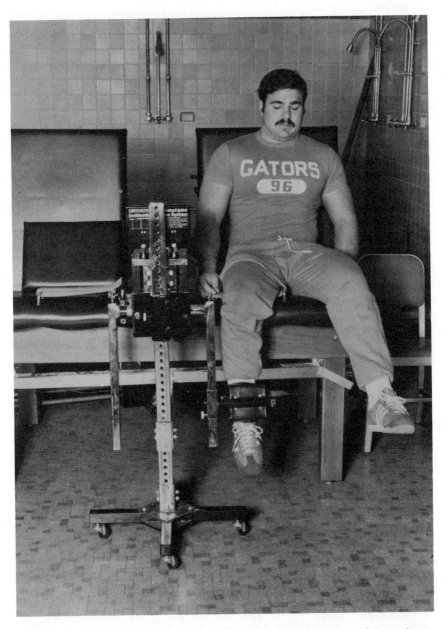

Isokinetic resistance is based on friction...which, by its nature, does not provide the back pressure required for stretching. In fact, the makers of isokinetic exercise devices point to this actual fault with apparent pride...hoping, I suppose, to give the impression that a major fault is actually an asset.

And in the third area, the *Nautilus* group improved more than twenty times as much as the conventional group, more than a 2,000 percent increase.

And, at the same time, while greatly improving their flexibility...the *Nautilus* trained subjects also increased in strength an average of nearly 60 percent, in only six weeks, as a result of only seventeen brief workouts...a total training time of approximately eight hours.

So it is obvious that properly conducted strength training will increase both strength and flexibility...and will do so rapidly.

And while it might be supposed that more training would have produced even better results...in fact, quite the opposite is true. Brief training is far more than a mere possibility...for best results, brief training is an absolute requirement.

For the purpose of increasing strength, a high intensity of work is beyond any question the single most important factor. And, given a truly high intensity of work, you literally cannot stand a large amount of training.

High-intensity exercise is required to stimulate growth...but it will also make deep inroads into your recovery ability, so it should not be overdone. No more than three high-intensity workouts should ever be performed within a period of a week, and no single workout should last much longer than thirty minutes.

Multiple sets are neither necessary nor desirable. One properly performed high-intensity set of each exercise is all that is required to provide a maximum degree of growth stimulation. Additional sets will merely make unnecessary inroads into your recovery ability...and similar to the effects of additional training may well prevent growth.

Illustrations 3-6 show that important differences exist between exercises performed for the same stated purpose. They also demonstrate that a proper style of performance can also provide an important difference.

Notice the enormous range of movement provided by the pullover machine (illustration 6) and compare this with the very limited range of movement involved in a pulldown exercise (illustration 5). Yet both exercises are performed for the same stated purpose: to develop the major muscles of the torso.

The pulldown exercise involves resistance over a range of movement of only about 120 degrees...and does not involve any actual stretching, or resistance in the fully contracted finishing position, which is never reached in this exercise.

In contrast, the pullover machine provides resistance over a range of movement in excess of 280 degrees. It involves stretching for even the most flexible athlete, and it has resistance in the fully contracted, finishing position. The pullover machine provides proper full-range exercise for the torso muscles. It is the only exercise that does.

Flexibility as a Result of Exercise

The use of such proper full-range exercises will increase flexibility, whiie simultaneously increasing strength throughout a full range of possible movement...and nothing else will.

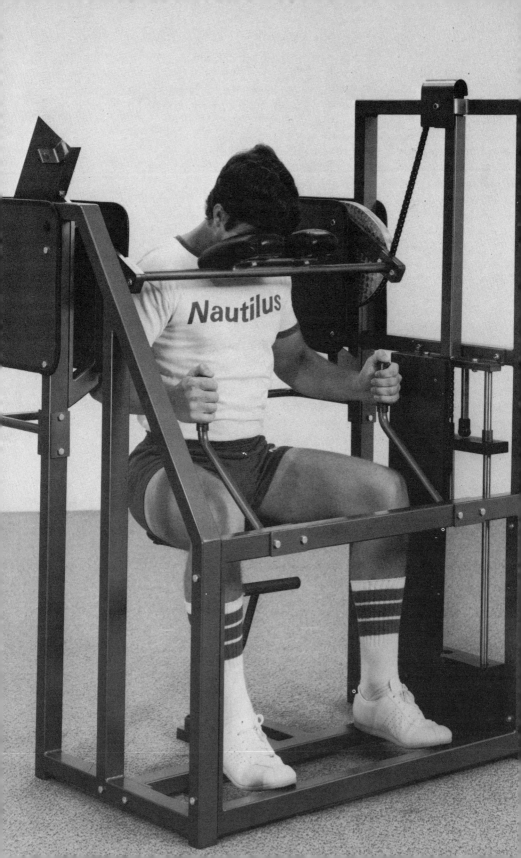

19
Increasing Neck Strength...
For the Prevention of Injury

By Arthur Jones

Neck injuries are the most common cause of death in football...but the number of fatal accidents comes nowhere close to indicating the actual extent of the problem. A far larger number of football players are injured to an important but lesser degree. One recent study stated that approximately ninety percent of all football players who are engaged in the sport for a period of several years will sustain permanent damage to the neck.

Injuries to the neck will continue to occur so long as football is played, regardless of what steps are taken in the direction of protective measures...but simple logic makes it obvious that a stronger neck is less likely to be injured in any given situation. So increasing the muscular strength and size of the neck is a long step in the direction of safety.

Unfortunately, until recently no really practical method existed for exercising the muscles of the neck; but that is a problem that no longer exists. Simple, practical and very productive equipment now exists for the rapid development of all of the important muscular structures of the neck.

During a recently conducted research program, eighteen subjects increased the carefully measured strength of their necks an average of 91.92 percent in a period of exactly six weeks...as a result of only twelve neck workouts of approximately eight minutes each.

These subjects were first trained on three new types of neck machines for a period of two weeks, and the progress produced during this initial two week period was not recorded. Then at the start of their third week of training, all subjects had their neck strength carefully measured on a tensiometer. Neck strength was measured in four directions: to the front, to the rear, and to both sides. The total of the four resulting figures was used as a starting score.

Then, exactly six weeks and twelve workouts later, the subjects were again tested on the tensiometer in the same manner. The results showed an average increase in neck strength for each of the eighteen subjects of 91.92 percent.

Since we did not test the subjects during the initial two weeks of training in order to avoid the so-called learning effect, it is impossible to say exactly what increase was produced during the entire eight weeks of training; but it was obvious to all observers that a large, if precisely unknown, increase in neck strength occurred during the first two weeks as well. One subject, for example, increased his neck measurement three-eighths of an inch from the first workout. Not the temporary increase of muscular "pump" but a permanent increase of actual muscular growth. Temporary muscular pump averaged well in excess of a full inch, and exceeded two inches in some cases.

These subjects trained only twice weekly, performing one set of each of seven exercises, utilizing three neck machines...a Nautilus 4-Way Neck machine...a Nautilus Rotary Neck machine...and a Nautilus Neck and Shoulder machine. These machines, in combination, provide proper full-range exercise for all seven functions of the neck muscles...1) anterior flexion...2) posterior extension...3) lateral flexion to the right...4) lateral flexion to the left...5) rotation to the right...6) rotation to the left...and 7) elevation of the shoulders.

During each of the two weeky workouts, the subjects performed only one set of approximately twelve repetitions of each of five exercises and one set of six repetitions of each of the other two exercises. Each entire workout averaged less than eight minutes.

The first exercise was a set of twelve repetitions of anterior flexion performed in a 4-Way Neck machine...immediately followed by a set of twelve repetitions of posterior extension in the same machine...followed by a set of twelve repetitions of lateral flexion to the right, still in the same machine...and then twelve repetitions of lateral flexion to the left, again in the same machine.

Having completed the first four exercises, all of which were performed in the 4-Way Neck machine, the subjects then moved immediately to the Rotary Neck machine for the next two exercises...rotation to the right and rotation to the left. These two exercises were performed in a negative-only style. Only six repetitions of each exercise were used.

The final exercise was one set of twelve repetitions performed using a Nautilus Neck and Shoulder machine.

During five of the seven exercises (the exceptions were the exercises on the Rotary Neck machine), the work was done in a normal fashion involving both positive and negative work. The resistance was lifted by the action of the neck muscles in a smooth and steady fashion, with absolutely nothing in the way of sudden movement or jerking. Upon reaching the top position of

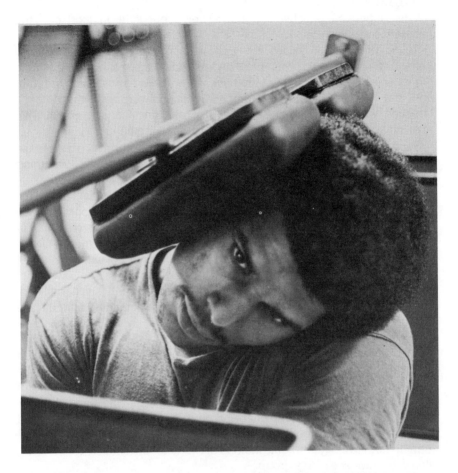

Injuries to the neck will continue to occur so long as football is played, regardless of what steps are taken in the direction of protective measures...but simple logic makes it obvious that a stronger neck is less likely to be injured in any given situation. So increasing the muscular strength and size of the neck is a long step in the direction of safety.

full muscular contraction, the subjects paused and held that position for approximately one second...and then slowly and smoothly lowered the weight back down to the starting position.

When it became possible to perform twelve repetitions in good form, the resistance was increased.

In the other two exercises, the work was performed in a negative-only fashion. While the head was forcefully rotated by the machine to the right, the muscles on the left side of the neck were worked by resisting the rotation, and vice versa. Six negative-only repetitions were performed in each direction, with a maximum possible level of resistance constantly regulated in exact accordance with the requirements of the moment.

Such a complete neck workout can easily be performed in five minutes or a bit less. In practice, however, the subjects usually required something more than seven minutes of elapsed time for a full neck workout, primarily because they usually did not move from one machine to the next as rapidly as they should. Thus, it is easily possible to produce full development of all of the neck muscles as a result of only ten minutes of weekly training...but in practice you can expect an average subject to devote approximately fifteen minutes to such training weekly. The training will consist of two workouts of about seven and a half minutes each.

All of the above mentioned subjects trained under supervised conditions, and part of the resulting increases in neck strength should be attributed to the supervision, which assured close attention to the style of performance of all exercises.

Another group of sixteen subjects trained in exactly the same fashion with only two exceptions... they trained three times weekly instead of twice weekly, and they were not supervised during their workouts. Members of this group increased an average of 56.72 percent within the same six week period, as a result of eighteen brief workouts. So the results were very good even without supervision...and there is strong evidence to indicate that performing three weekly workouts instead of two actually reduced the resulting strength increases in this group.

Two other groups of twelve subjects (twenty-four subjects altogether) also trained in an unsupervised fashion; with one group performing only two weekly workouts and the other group performing three weekly workouts. Similar to the groups with sixteen subjects, the twice-a-week group also produced somewhat better results.

In this comparison, both groups trained for a total of only four weeks, with no pre-test training...so one group trained a total of only eight times, while the other group performed a total of twelve workouts. The twice-a-week group increased neck strength an average of 41.6 percent from only eight workouts...while the three-times-a-week, group increased an average of 39.8 percent from four more workouts.

Thus, the value of supervision is obvious, but it also appears that an extra, third weekly workout is of no value and may actually reduce the rate of strength increase.

At least one other result of this research program was also rather surprising. At the start of the program we knew that the weakest of the four neck-strength tests was the one that measured anterior flexion, the strength of the muscles of the front of the neck. We also knew that the strongest was a measurement of posterior extension, measuring the strength of the muscles of the back of the neck.

But this ratio of front to back strength changed during the course of the eight week program. The frontal neck muscles increased in strength at a faster rate than the other neck muscles, perhaps because they had been the most neglected of a generally neglected group of muscles. With a longer program of proper neck training, the author would not be surprised to see this ratio change to the extent that the frontal neck muscles become the strongest.

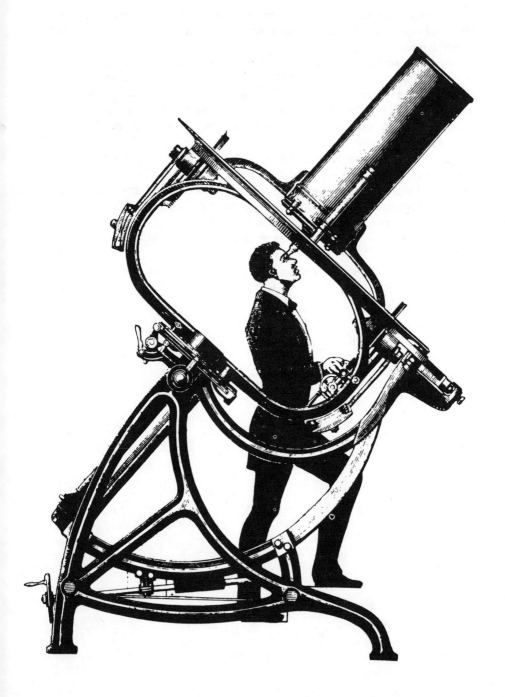

20
The Future of Exercise
An Opinion

By Arthur Jones

Now that the medical profession has finally, if belatedly, recognized at least part of the potentially great value of exericse, it behooves everybody to approach the subject on a logical basis. If not, then the doctors now becoming interested in sports medicine will be forced to learn the hard way, by repeating many of the mistakes that others have already made.

An enormous quantity of literature exists on the subject of exercise, for those whom have time to read it...but if so, where do you start, who do you believe, what do you believe? The presently existing controversy is that we might well be far better off with absolutely nothing in the way of literature on the subject of exercise; then perhaps the whole issue could be approached on rational grounds.

Millions of people have already devoted literally billions of hours to trial and error experimentation, so experience is certainly not one of the factors that is lacking...but in fact, very little of any value seems to have been gained by all that experience. On the contrary, myths and supersitions still abound; while the simple facts remain largely ignored, frequently even unsuspected.

And what are the facts? The point of primary importance is the simple fact that functional ability is improved by proper exercise. But, then, just what is proper exercise?

Logically, proper exercise can only be defined as the minimum amount of exercise that will produce the desired result. Anything in excess of that minimum is by definition unnecessary, therefore illogical...and possibly contraproductive.

The Future of Exercise - An Opinion

Probably the most damaging misconception in the field of exercise is the widespread, almost universal tendency to equate quantity with quality. This is a seemingly natural tendency, and therefore understandable...but this tendency runs squarely in the face of the facts. It utterly ignores the unavoidable interrelationship of intensity of work and amount of work.

There is an obvious but unmeasurable threshold of intensity...below which no amount of exercise will stimulate the improvement of functional ability. But just how do we define intensity of work? And how can we ever be sure that an unknown, even unmeasurable, level has been reached?

Intensity of work is a relative factor having absolutely no relationship to the amount of work. It can best be defined, I think, as the percentage of momentary ability. In which case it can be measured accurately at only two possible levels, 100 percent and zero...when you are working as hard as momentarily possible, or when you are doing absolutely nothing.

A very brief experiment is all that is required to prove that a zero level of intensity will quickly produce both muscular atrophy and a loss in cardiovascular ability. Obviously, a level of work somewhat above zero is obviously called for.

An even briefer experiment will also prove that you cannot work at a level of 100 percent for more than a few seconds. The unavoidable conclusion is that we must work somewhere between the only levels of intensity that are measurable. But where? At what level? For how long? How often?

Those are the questions that have produced the current widespread controversy in the field of exercise. Practical answers to these qustions already exist but the answers still remain largely unknown, or even denied.

Unknown by whom? By the vast majority of doctors now beginning to become interested in sports medicine. Denied by whom? By a wide array of conflicting commercial interests, and even by most of the supposed experts in the field of exercise, the research scientists.

The future of exercise depends upon the resolution of the questions now being so hotly debated. Until and unless something approaching a general consensus is reached, the existing confusion will simply be compounded.

Additional research may or may not be the answer; but if the existing literature resulting from previous research in the field offers any reasonable criteria for judgment, then I think we can look forward to at least another century of confusion, missed opportunities, and largely wasted effort.

Or it may even turn out worse; the present confusion could easily lead the medical profession, as a whole, into an almost outright rejection of exercise. And if so, once having been rejected, many centuries could pass before exercise will even be afforded the courtesy of another look. In which case, the loss to everybody would be enormous.

While future improvements in existing equipment are almost certain, the primary problem exists elsewhere. Very good results can be produced by

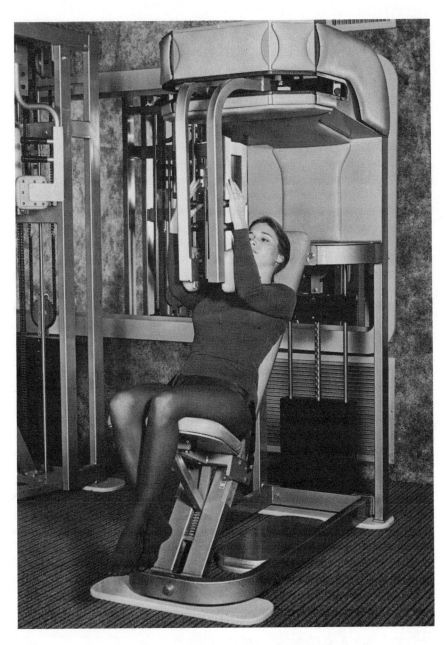

Logically, proper exercise can only be defined as the minimum amount of exercise that will produce the desired result. Anything in excess of that minimum is by definition unnecessary, therefore illogical...and possibly contra-productive.

the proper use of a wide variety of exercise equipment that is already available. The real problem, as I see it, is getting people to utilize the existing equipment properly.

The mere existence of equipment that is capable of producing good results is apparently not enough; in an ideal world it might be, but in the real world it isn't...most people seemingly need equipment that literally cannot be used in any manner except a proper manner. If it can be misused, it usually will be misused.

Enter the computer. And with the aid of a computer, this is the way I see the future of exercise. Five years into the future? Ten years? I don't know, but coming; perhaps for no better reason than the fact that it is now possible, and anything that can happen probably will happen. Or maybe it will happen out of sheer economic necessity, since truly widespread utilization of proper exercise is not economically feasible under currently existing circumstances. Since proper supervision of exercise is prohibitively expensive already and steadily increasing, such supervision must come from a non-human source, from a machine, a computer. And it will.

Enter the gym of the future, pull your pre-programmed plastic card out of the file and insert it into a slot in the machine...and from that moment on, the machine will tell you exactly what to do, how to do it, and how often to do it. And keep an accurate permanent record of what you actually do.

As soon as your card is inserted your number will appear on the first of several exercise machines. This machine will be instantly and automatically set for you with careful consideration for all of your individual requirements: your existing strength level, your degree of flexibility, your cardiovascular ability, your age, your medical history, and any other important considerations.

The level of resistance? Whatever you require at that point in time; but the machine itself will actually provide no resistance at all. You will be the source of your own resistance, providing resistance for the concentric exercise of one limb by the eccentric work of the bilateral limb. The results will come from an almost silent form of exercise which has many advantages over conventional forms of exercise with their external sources of resistance, weights or friction.

In effect, using a leg press exercise as an example, your right leg would provide the resistance required to work your left leg, and vice versa. Upon seating yourself in the leg press machine, you will find two separate foot pads located precisely at the mid-range of possible movement. This makes it very easy to enter the machine, since you are not required to wedge yourself into position against a force of resistance.

So entry is quick, easy, and safe...a consideration of no small importance.

To start the exercise, it is merely necessary to press against one of the foot pads, thereby straightening that leg; whereupon, as one leg straightens, the opposite foot pads will be forced back towards you and your other leg will be required to bend.

Kindly note; I did not say that your other leg would be *forced* to bend...instead, I said it would be *required* to bend, the difference being significant.

The leg that is being straightened will be working concentrically. It will be performing positive work. The leg that is bending will be working eccentrically, performing negative work. In the realm of muscular work at least, negative is far stronger than positive. The net result is that you would find it simply impossible to force one leg to bend by the use of the straightening force available in the other leg; not unless a gross imbalance in bilateral strength existed.

So the positive working limb cannot force the negative working limb to do anything. Instead, the negative working limb must permit movement of the positive working limb.

The result is that you are literally provided with an infinite source of resistance, as much as you can handle while working at a 100 percent level of intensity and more...or as little as you want...or anything in between.

Disregarding a slight and unimportant amount of unavoidable mechanical friction, the level of force will be exactly equal in both the negative and positive parts of the work. If your right leg is pushing with a force of 200 pounds, then an exactly equal level of force will be pushing back against your left leg.

In such a machine, it is easily possible to make every positive movement a maximum-possible effort involving an intensity of work of 100 percent...but in practice, doing so is neither necessary nor desirable. Instead, the first several repetitions should be performed at an intensity well below 100 percent...for several reasons: to greatly reduce the chances of injury, to gradually warm up and lubricate the working muscles and moving joints, and to pre-exhaust the muscles so that one or two repetitions can be performed at the end of the exercise while keeping the actual force at a relatively low level.

And just how do we know how hard to push? The machine will tel l us; if we push too hard, the machine will tell us, instantly...if we don't push hard enough, the machine will tell us.

If we push exactly as hard as we should, then the actual amount of force produced by one leg will remain constant throughout most of the exercise; and when it becomes momentarily impossible to produce that level of force, then it is time to stop.

But while the actual force will remain constant in such an exercise, the level of intensity will increase from repetition to repetition until, at the end of a properly performed set of twelve repetitions, the muscles would be working at a level of intensity of 100 percent.

And don't now jump to a hasty conclusion. Instead of being somehow different in that regard from conventional exercises, a moment of consideration will make it obvious that exactly the same thing happens in all conventional exercises if more than one repetition is performed.

Only one repetition of 100 percent intensity is possible in any conventional exercise, regardless of the number of repetitions performed. Because, if the first repetition is of 100 percent intensity, then it will also be the last, the only one possible. It is possible to stop an exercise well short of an intensity of 100 percent...but it is utterly impossible to continue an exercise after the performance of one repetition of 100 percent intensity.

The resistance involved in the exercises of the future of the gym I am discussing will not be isokinetic in nature; instead, such a form of bilateral, self-generated resistance is called infimetric. Similar to an isokinetic form of resistance, it is easily possible to perform several repetitions of 100 percent intensity while using infimetric exercises. Doing so is neither necessary nor desirable.

The ten basic requirements for a truly full-range exercise are as follows...1) direct resistance...2) rotary form resistance...3) automatically variable resistance...4) balanced resistance...5) positive work...6) negative work...7) stretching...8) pre-stretching...9) unlimited speed of movement...10) resistance in a position of full muscular contraction. All of these requirements will be provided in most of the exercise machines used in the gym of the future.

Seated in the first exercise machine; press out with the right leg, smoothly and fairly slowly...the left leg is simultaneously pushed into a bent position of muscular stretch. Pause, stretch a bit more, and then, taking advantage of the pre-stretch reflex, immediately press out with the left leg while the previously straight right leg starts to bend. Continue for a total of approximately ten positive repetitions for each leg, while never changing the input for force; then, having momentarily reduced your starting strength level by the earlier submaximal repetitions for each leg...making each of these last four positive movements a maximum effort, utilizing 100 percent intensity.

Danger? Little, if any; almost none insofar as a danger of pulling a muscle or its connective tissue is concerned...because, by the end of the exercise, you literally aren't stronger enough to hurt yourself if you maintain anything even approaching good form. Regardless of the fact that the momentary intensity is then 100 percent, it nevertheless is also true that the level of force remains relatively low throughout the exercise and is actually at its lowest point during the final four movements. High-intensity, but low-force, exercise...productive and safe.

Such exercises already exist. The only thing really lacking in order to build the gym of the future right now is linking a variety of these machines to a computer; but computers also exist...so the marriage will occur and is already occurring.

The machines of the future gym won't make you exercise properly, noth-

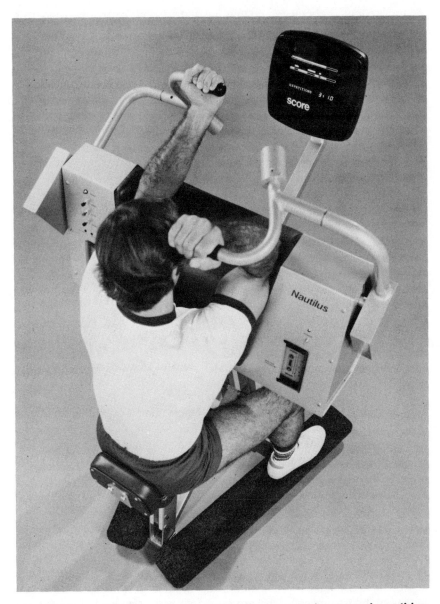

The machines of the future gym won't make you exercise properly, nothing can do that...nobody can do that. All that anybody or anything can do is make it possible for you to exercise properly, and then encourage you to exercise properly, tell you when you are doing something right, and when you are doing something wrong; and the machine can do all those things, and do them far better than any human supervisor.

ing can do that...nobody can do that. All that anybody or anything can do is make it possible for you to exercise properly, and then encourage you to exercise properly, tell you when you are doing something right, and when you are doing something wrong; and the machine can do all of those things, and do them far better than any human supervisor.

Additionally, the machine can do many things that no human can do like keeping an instant and exact record of your actual workouts...automatically, instantly, and correctly changing your workouts when they need changing. Sensing and reacting to any reasonable number of physiological factors, pulse, blood pressure, and other factors.

And what will such a facility cost? In hard figures, that remains an impossible question at the moment. In a practical sense, however, the price will undoubtedly be far lower than the present cost of properly supervised exercise. If for no other reason than the simple fact that one supervisor could easily and simultaneously supervise the workouts of several hundred individuals.

And what will be the results of such exercise? Any kind and degree of results that can now be produced by any type of exercise...increased strength cardiovascular ability...rehabilitation following certain types of illness...or a program designed merely to maintain a previously built level of strength, flexibiity or cardiovascular ability.

The machines can be computer programmed for any purpose; but perhaps of greatest importance, a machine won't lose interest in the subjects working under its supervision.

The most difficult, and certainly the most widespread problem at the present state of the art seems to be the one of motivation. In a practical sense, it is difficult to get people to perform their exercises properly. If both the form and intensity of work are proper, then exercise is capable of producing surprising results in a short span of time. There, however, seems to be a natural tendency on the part of most people to permit a rapid deterioration in the style of performance, or form...as well as a tendency to gradually reduce the intensity of exercise without even being aware that such is occurring.

The design of most presently existing exercise equipment makes such problems almost inevitable; the problems are inherent...but they can be solved. Both problems, poor form and lowered intensity, result from a desire to show progress; thus, under the mistaken impression that they are thereby improving at a faster rate, most people quickly start changing the form or intensity of their exercises...and are encouraged in this direction by the fact that doing so increases the amount of resistance they can handle, makes it possible for them to lift more weight. Or, in fact, makes it possible for them to throw more weight; because, by that point, they are no longer lifting the weight; instead, they are throwing the weight.

No increase in resistance is meaningful unless the form remains unchanged, and no amount of exercise will produce good results if the form is not good. But just what is good form in exercise?

The answer to this question depends upon the purpose of the exercise. Developing muscular stength requires certain factors that are not necessary if you are interested only in increasing cardiovascular ability...although, in fact, properly performed strength exercises unavoidably will increase cardiovascular ability as well as strength.

During a large-scale research program that we conducted in cooperation with the physical education department of the United States Military Academy at West Point, during April and May of 1975, it was clearly demonstrated that properly performed strength exercises in fact do have very meaningful effects upon cardiovascular ability. For example, in one such test of cardiovascular fitness, the two mile run, our Wholebody Group of 19 subjects reduced their time by an average of 88 seconds as a result of only six weeks of strength training. While a control group of 15 subjects reduced their average time in the two mile run by an average of only 20 seconds during the same six-week period.

Both groups were composed of varsity football players. Since both groups were involved in spring football practice during the period of the experiment, the improvement shown by the control group can be attributed to the training involved in spring football practice. And, obviously, approximately 20 seconds of the improvement shown by the experimental group must also be attributed to spring football practice, but the remaining improvement of 68 seconds was a direct result of the strength testing. While it is certainly possible to improve strength while doing little or nothing to improve cardiovascular ability, it is neither necessary nor desirable to do so. This point was clearly and decisively demonstrated by the West Point study.

During the same study, the Wholebody Group of subjects increased their neck strength an average of 91.92 percent...in a period of only six weeks, as a result of twelve very brief workouts. While a matched control group improved its neck strength an average of only 27.84 percent as a result of training that formed part of spring football practice during the same span of six weeks.

Obviously, the form, or style of performance, of proper exercise depends upon the purpose of the training; although, in fact, certain basic rules should be applied to any exercise performed for any purpose.

But the gym of the future will provide for the utilization of any worthwhile style of performance, for any purpose. And, of far greater importance, it will prevent certain dangerous styles of performance. While it may not literally force you to train right, it will prevent you from using many of the dangerous and non-productive styles of training that are so common today. And, if you don't train right, you and your supervisor will both be clearly aware of it...instantly.

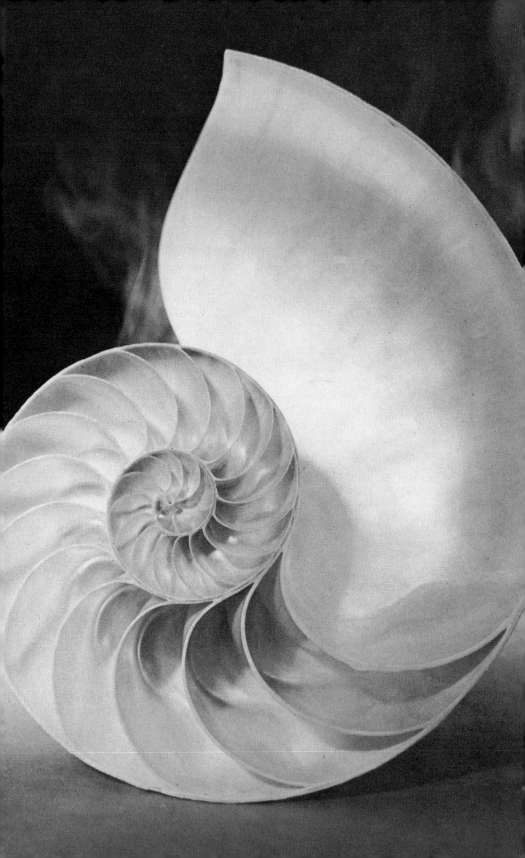

PART B

NAUTILUS TRAINING:
PRINCIPLES AND TECHNIQUES

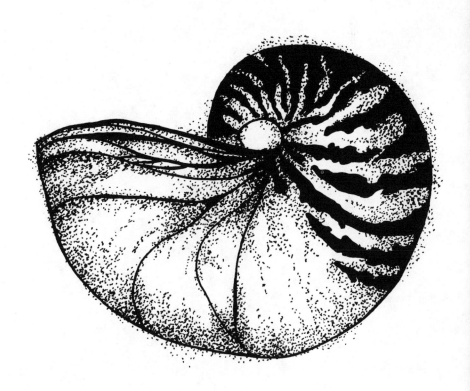

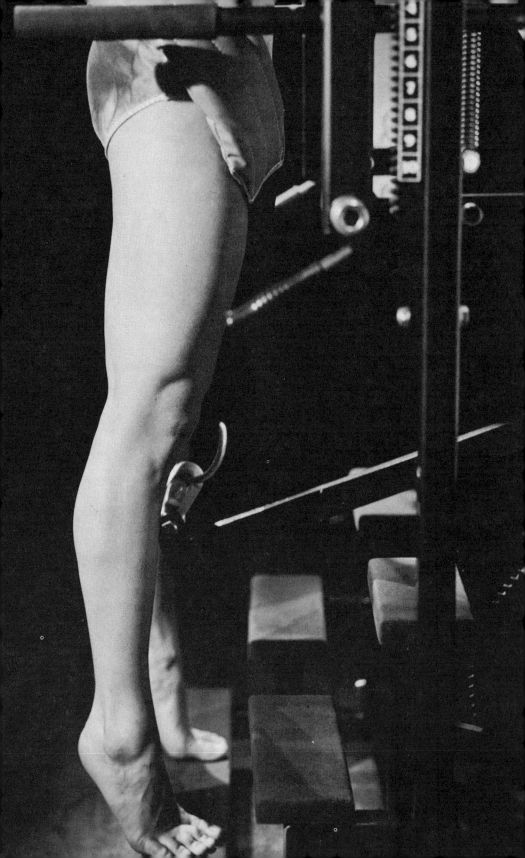

21

Strength Training Principles*

By Ellington Darden, Ph.D.
Director of Research
Nautilus Sports/Medical Industries, Inc.

Proper strength training will benefit any athlete, young or old. As a result, he will be stronger, faster, more flexible, more enduring, and far less likely to suffer injury.

Muscular strength is one of the most important factors to an athlete. Why? Primarily, because it provides the power behind every movement. Secondly, because of the role it plays in protecting the athlete from injury. Not only do stronger muscles enable an athlete to run faster, throw and kick farther, and move more efficiently; but they also provide increased joint stability—whether it be the ankle, knee, hip, shoulder, neck, elbow, or wrist.

Many high school, college, and professional athletic teams have strength training programs of some form or fashion. The results that are gained, however, from this vast amount of training time and effort fall far short of what they should be. Most athletes lightly scratch the surface of the potentially great value of strength training. The problems seem to stem from **faulty training techniques**, techniques that not only limit the results, but contribute to injuries...and a **lack of understanding** built on a long list of handed down myths and superstitions.

What is the right way to build strength? How often should you train? Which methods should you use? What exercises are best? And, generally speaking, how can you distinguish between fact and folly?

This chapter was written to answer these questions and provide you with some basic guidelines for use in establishing sound strength training programs. Six basic principles of strength training will be discussed. Following each principle are sub-principles which in turn are followed by the implications of these guidelines. I might add that these guidelines can be used with Nautilus, Universal, or conventional equipment.

*Reprinted from *Strength Training by the Experts* (Daniel P. Riley, editor) by permission of the publisher, Leisure Press, West Point, New York.

1.0 Strength training must be progressive; you should constantly attempt to increase the repetitions or resistance in every workout.

Strength cannot be increased by the mere repetition of things that are already easy. You must constantly attempt the momentarily impossible. Attempting the momentarily impossible causes the body to resort to its reserve ability. Forcing the body to use this reserve ability is an important factor in stimulating a muscle to get stronger.

Sub-principle 1.1   In general, best results will occur if repetitions are kept in the 8 to 12 range.

If you perform less than 6 repetitions of an exercise, little inroads will be made into your reserve ability. On the other hand, if you perform over 15 repetitions, you will probably fail from a lack of oxygen, rather than from having reached a point of actual muscular failure. Once again you would not be working inside the level of your reserve ability. Greater inroads can be made into your reserve ability, if you work with resistance you can handle from 8 to 12 repetitions.

Sub-principle 1.2   When you perform 12 repetitions—or more—that is the signal to increase the resistance (by approximately 5%) in that exercise at the time of the next workout.

Empirical evidence has shown that optimum strength gains for the skeletal muscles occur when the exercise is at least 40 seconds in duration, but not more than about 70 seconds. Therefore, if you performed 10 repetitions of a given exercise, simple division reveals that each repetition should take from four to seven seconds.

Sub-principle 1.3   Never terminate a set simply because a certain number of repetitions have been completed; a set is properly finished only when additional movement is utterly impossible.

Under ideal conditions, your progress should be steady and consistent. Most training, however, does not take place under ideal conditions. As a result, strength increases are often up and down. For example, over a two-week period of time, the number of strict repetitions that you perform of a curl with a 100-pound barbell might look like the following: 8, 8, 9, 11, 10, 13. Regardless of the guide number of repetitions you're attempting to perform, you should curl until you cannot bend your arms. But, you should only record the number of repetitions you performed in perfect form.

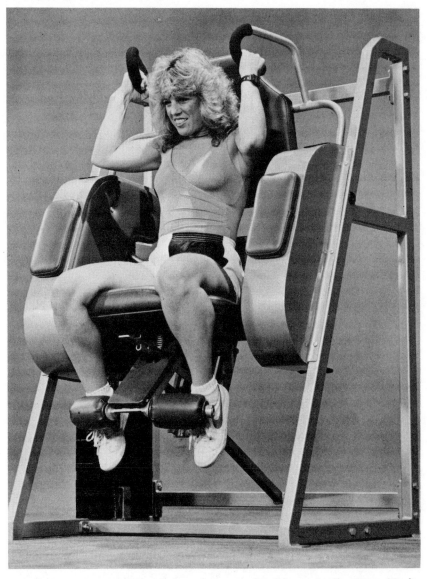

Strength training must be progressive; you should constantly attempt to increase the repetitions or resistance in every workout.

'Sub-principle 1.4 Training should be done to build strength, not demonstrate it; therefore, how much you can lift for one repetition should be avoided.

Lifting maximum weights, as in weight lifting, certainly requires strength. But it also requires skill, a skill that must be developed by the practice of lifting maximum weights, and a skill that is of no value for any other purpose except lifting weights (competitive weight lifting). In fact, this skill is actually dangerous. Why? Because it exposes the muscles and connective tissue to a level of force that may cause injury. An injury will result when the forces involved in suddenly lifting (or more correctly, "throwing") a weight exceed the structural integrity of a muscle, tendon, or joint. All the worthwhile results of strength training can be produced with little or no risk of injury by using 8 to 12 repetitions in each exercise.

Implications. The cornerstone of strength training is progression, or constantly trying to increase the workload each training session. The only practical way to be progressive is by using barbells, dumbbells, or weight machines (e.g., Universal and Nautilus).

It is important to keep accurate records on your progress. The weight and the number of perfect repetitions should be written down immediately after each exercise. Also the time spent on each workout should be recorded.

Best results are usually produced when a set involves at least 8 repetitions and not more than 12 repetitions. Single repetition, maximum possible attempts, should be avoided at all costs...unless you're a competitive weight lifter. If you're not willing to perform actually progressive exercise (and it is certainly not an easy style of training), then you will never produce the final results that could have been produced.

2.0 The building of strength is related to the intensity of exercise: the higher the intensity, the better the muscles are stimulated.

Working men commonly perform enormous amounts of work, with very little in the way of strength increases as a result of their efforts. Careful research has established the cause and effect relationship involved in this situation; greatly increased muscular strength is not produced by common labor because the intensity of muscular contraction is low.

The "overload principle" is required for the production of significant increases in muscular strength. The muscles must be exposed to a load that produces high-intensity contraction.

Intensity of contraction has probably been best defined as percentage of momentary ability. When a muscle is producing as much pulling force as it is momentarily capable of doing, then maximum intensity of contraction is involved.

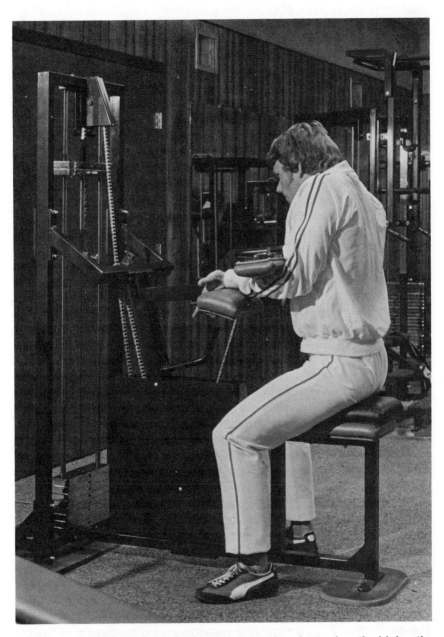

The building of strength is related to the intensity of exercise: the higher the intensity, the better the muscles are simulated.

Sub-principle 2.1 Individual muscle fibers perform on an "all or nothing" basis; only the number of fibers that are actually required to move a particular amount of resistance are involved in any movement.

In effect, a fiber is working as hard as possible—or not at all. A movement against light resistance does not involve a small amount of work on the part of all of the fibers in the muscles contributing to this movement. Instead, only a few fibers are involved—the minimum number of fibers that are required to move the imposed resistance—and the remainder of the fibers are not involved. But the fibers that are working, are working as hard as possible—as hard as possible at that moment.

One individual fiber may be involved in each of several repetitions in a set of an exercise, but it will not contribute an equal amount of power to each repetition. The fiber will always be working as hard as possible—or not at all—but its strength will decline with each additional repetition.

Thus, in practice, a set might involve a number of fibers in much the following fashion. The first repetition involves 10 fibers, with each fiber contributing 10 "units of power" to the movement. The second repetition involves the same 10 fibers, which then contribute only 9 units of power each, and one previously uninvolved fiber (an eleventh fiber, a fresh fiber) that contributes 10 units of power, bringing the total power production up to the same level as that involved in the first repetition. The third repetition might involve the same initially used 10 fibers, with each of them now contributing only 8.1 units of power, plus the eleventh fiber that was used previously only during the second repetition, and which now contibutes 9 units of power, plus a twelfth fiber, a fresh fiber that is involved for the first time only during the third repetition and contributes 10 units of power.

Each of the first three repetitions, therefore, would result in exactly the same amount of power production. And all of the involved fibers would always be contributing to the limit of their momentary ability. The fibers, however, would not be contributing equally, and the actual number of involved fibers would change from repetition to repetition.

If the set was ended at that point, then little or nothing in the way of growth stimulating was produced—because none of the fibers was worked very hard, and because there were still unused fibers in reserve.

In order to produce significant growth stimulation, the set must be continued to a point where as many as possible of the available fibers have been involved—and where at least some of the fibers have been worked to a point of total failure.

Sub-principle 2.2 A set that is terminated prior to the point of failure will not involve the maximum available muscle fibers.

Sub-principle 2.3 A slight decrease in the intensity of effort will cause a disproportionate reduction in the results.

Sub-principle 2.4 It is impossible to measure intensity of effort less than maximum possible (100%) effort.

Exercise below a certain percentile of the momentary existing level of ability will produce no increases in muscular size and strength, regardless of the amount of exercise. There seems to be a definite "break-over" point, a point below which growth will not be stimulated, and above which growth will be stimulated. Having passed above that break-over point in the required intensity of exercise, the results seem to increase in a geometric fashion.

It may be that somewhat less than 100% of the momentary possible level of intensity is all that is required to produce maximum growth stimulation. But even if that might be the case, it is obvious that any such difference in the required intensity of effort and an outright 100% intensity of effort is of no significance.

And even if it was proven that all that was required for maximum possible growth stimulating was a level of intensity of, for example, 95% of momentary ability, just how would you propose to use such information? How would you actually know if you were working at a level of 95%, instead of 90%, or 85%? How would you measure it?

But you can measure 100%, simply by performing each exercise to a point of utter failure.

Sub-principle 2.5 In order to obtain maximum possible intensity of exercise, you must be closely supervised and "pushed."

If left to their own devices, most people will not train properly. Human nature being as it is, all of us (to a greater or lesser extent) will both consciously and unconsciously do almost everything possible to make an exercise easier. Observe any group of athletes training without supervision and you will see all types of "cheating" movements mixed in with a consistent "stopping short of failure." Exercise should be made harder, not easier—and when you make exercise harder, it must be properly supervised—every repetition of every exercise of every workout.

Implications. High intensity of muscular contraction is the single most important factor in exercises performed for the purpose of increasing muscular strength. It is very easy to slip back into a much easier style of training, frequently without being aware that you are doing so. Therefore, for maximum possible results, someone that knows what they're doing should supervise each of your workouts.

3.0 Each repetition should be performed with special attention given to a slow speed of movement, a great range of movement, and pre-stretching of the involved muscles.

Sub-principle 3.1   The speed of movement must not be too fast and not too slow.

If you performed a barbell exercise at various speeds while standing on a force plate connected to a recorder, you could clearly see the difference between slow and fast repetitions. Repetitions performed in a slow, smooth manner apply steady force throughout the entire movement. Fast repetitions apply force to only a small portion (at the start and at the end) of the movement.

Sub-principle 3.2   Special attention should be given to the lowering portion (eccentric contraction) of all exercises.

Research has shown that for building muscular strength, lowering the resistance is more important than raising the resistance. A good rule of thumb is...it should take 2 seconds to raise a weight and 4 seconds (or twice as long) to lower the same weight. All in all, it should take about one minute to complete a set of 10 repetitions.

Sub-principle 3.3   "Jerky" movements should be avoided at all costs.

When a weight is jerked or thrown, a large amount of force (usually from three to four times the actual weight) is directed on the muscles and joints. This is both dangerous and unproductive.

Sub-principle 3.4   The range of movement of each repetition should be as great as possible (from full extension to full contraction).

In order to contract, a muscle must produce movement. And in order to contract fully, a muscle must produce a full range of possible movement. If the movement resulting from muscular contraction is less than full range, then the entire length of the muscle is not involved in the work. In addition, prevention of injury is most likely where the muscles have been strengthened in every position and over a full range of possible movement.

Sub-principle 3.5   Each repetition should start from a pre-stretched position.

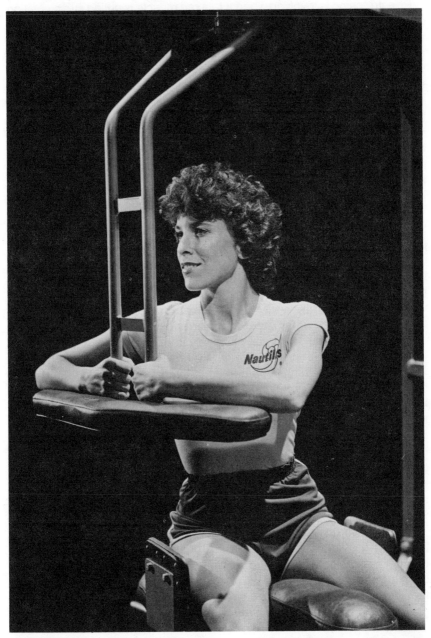

Each repetition should be performed with special attention given to slow speed of movement, a great range of movement, and pre-stretching of the involved muscles.

Pre-stretching is involved when a relaxed muscle is pulled into a position of increased tension prior to the start of contraction. Pre-stretching, properly applied, enables you to handle heavier weights and thus bring into action a greater percentage of your muscle mass during each repetition. For example, the weight should be lowered from the contracted position in a controlled manner until the bar is about one inch from the position of full extension. At that point, there should be a quick "twitch." Immediately following the quick "twitch," the movement should be slowed down in a controlled manner. The only rapid manner of the bar should be during the last portion of the lowering part of the repetition and the first part of the raising part of the repetition. The remaining portion of each repetition should always be performed slowly.

Implications. Many of you are involved or have been involved in some type of strength training program. Perhaps you've always performed fast, jerky repetitions, with little attention given to the lowering portion (eccentric contraction) or the movement. It is hard to break old habits. In fact, the act of breaking these old habits means that you must reduce the resistance in almost every exercise. It is important, therefore, to understand that...**lifting a weight is not enough, regardless of the amount of weight. How you lift a weight is a factor of far greater importance.**

Remember, it should take approximately 2 seconds in the raising part and 4 seconds in the lowering part of each exercise.

There are certain things you can do to intensify the lowering portion of some exercises. Two "spotters" can assist you in lifting the weight (a much heavier weight than you could normally lift yourself) and then allow you to lower the weight in a controlled fashion. Or, in a chinning and dipping movement, you can attach a 25-pound dumbbell to a belt around your waist, step up on a chair to the top position, and lower yourself very slowly (8-10 seconds).

With Universal or Nautilus machines, you can perform the movement in a slightly different manner. Raise the resistance with two limbs, and lower with only one limb. Raise with two, lower with the opposite.

As for pre-stretching in a strength training exercise, there is a thin line between (1) pre-stretching a muscle in the starting position and following through with the repetition in the proper form, and (2) pre-stretching a muscle in the starting position and throwing the resistance. The key points to remember are pre-stretch—move quickly—and then slow down. If in doubt, always perform a repetition **slower**, rather than faster.

Strength Training Principles

4.0 Exercises should be selected that involve the greatest range of movement of the major muscle groups.

First of all, a thorough mechanical analysis should be made to determine the muscle groups that are directly involved in your particular sport. Most sports require great strength in all muscle groups, with gymnastics and sprinting being possible exceptions. Once you determine the muscles that need to be strengthened, the next step is to select exercises that involve full-range movement (or as close to full-range movement as possible) for these muscles.

In order for an exercise to be full-range, there must be resistance throughout the movement, in the extended position, in the mid-range, and in the contracted position. Full-range movements are impossible with a barbell or a Universal machine in all but a few exercises: shoulder shrugs, standing calf raises, and wrist curls with the forearms on a declined surface. Full-range movements, however, are possible with a wide variety of Nautilus machines. The Nautilus machines that provide full-range exercise are as follows: hip and back, leg extension, leg curl, pullover, behind neck, rowing, double shoulder (primary movement), double chest (primary movement), neck and shoulder, 4-way neck, rotary neck, and several varieties of bicep curl and tricep extension machines.

If full-range resistance is impossible, as it will prove to be in most exercises, then select exercises that provide the greatest range of movement. For example, the full squat, stiff-legged deadlift, chin-up, parallel dip, press, and curl.

Sub-principle 4.1 Generally speaking, the greater the mass of the muscle involved, the greater the value of the exercise.

Using conventional equipment, the exercises that involve the greatest muscle mass are compound movements, or exercises that involve rotation of two or more joints. For example, the standing press (which involves movement around the elbow and shoulder joints) is a much better exercise than the tricep extension (which involves movement around the elbow).

Sub-principle 4.2 Do not try to improve a sport skill by devising a strength exercise that is similar to the skill.

This principle is the one most likely to be violated by both the experienced and inexperienced coach and athlete. An example should make this point clear.

Motor learning research indicates that learning a simple movement with a badminton racquet, such as hitting a bird against the wall, will impede the

221

learning (negative transfer) of an apparently similar skill, hitting a tennis ball against a wall. In both skills similar stimulus conditions are present: a racquet, an object to be hit, and a wall. However, the reponses required are different. In badminton, wrist action is very important, while in tennis the wrist should remain relatively stiff.

Similarly, practice at putting a 20-pound shot will not help an athlete to improve his 16-pound shot putting ability. In fact, it will probably confuse him. Punting or passing a five-pound football would be another step in the wrong direction—of course it would help if the athlete wanted to **learn how** to punt or pass a five-pound football.

Yet, thousands of coaches have their athletes perform arm and leg strengthening exercises in a manner that stimulates a skill (e.g., bench presses performed very rapidly for improving power in swinging a baseball bat, or jumping squats with dumbbells for improving jumping ability). To practice movements that are **nearly** the same as those of the task can not only be confusing, but it can be disastrous.

How, then, should an athlete strength train? He should select exercises that **do not** simulate the skills he desires to improve—exercises that are totally different in meaning, form, and method of execution. Exercises that involve no inter-task transfer...no positive transfer...no negative transfer.

Athletes should develop strength **generally** in all major muscle groups. Then, this general strength can be used to improve any specific ability that requires the contraction and extension of the strengthened muscles.

Anyone who has ever used a barbell is aware that the exercises provided by the use of such a piece of equipment are not full-range movements. At some points in most barbell exercises, there is no resistance at all—at the start of a curl, at the end of most forms of curling, at the top position in a squat or a press of any kind. If you can "lock out" under the weight in any position, then you do not have full-range resistance. In such a case you are providing exercise for only part of the muscles that you are trying to work.

Full-range resistance can only be provided by a machine that rotates on a common axis with the body part that is moved by the muscles being worked. When this requirement is met, then it becomes possible to provide exercise that actually exceeds the range-of-movement that is possible for most trainees. At this point in time, Nautilus sports/Medical Industries makes the only exercise machines that actually provide full-range exercise. Therefore, if you have access to Nautilus machines, be sure and use them. You will get faster and better results.

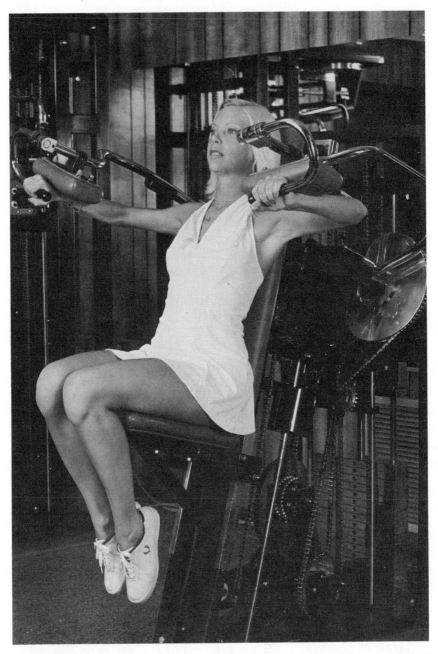

Exercises should be selected that involve the greatest range of movement of the major muscle groups.

Implications. The following exercises, grouped by muscle group and equipment, are applicable to most strength training programs:

Muscle Group	Barbells/Dumbbells	Universal Gym	Nautilus Machines
Buttocks/lower back	squat stiff-legged deadlift	leg press hyperextension	hip and back squat leg press
Quadriceps	squat	leg extension leg press	leg extension squat leg press
Hamstrings	squat	leg curl leg press	leg curl squat leg press
Calves	calf raise	toe press on leg press	calf raise on multi exercise toe press on leg press
Latissimus dorsi	bent-over rowing bent-armed pullover stiff-armed pullover	chin-up pulldown on lat machine	pullover behind neck torso/arm chin-up on multi exercise
Trapezius	shoulder shrug dumbbell shoulder shrug	shoulder shrug	neck and shoulder rowing torso

Muscle			
Deltoids	press press behind neck upright rowing forward raise side raise with dumbbells	seated press upright rowing	double shoulder • lateral raise • overhead press omni shoulder rowing torso
Pectoralis majors	bench press dumbbell flies	double chest parallel dip	• arm cross • decline press • parallel dip on multi exercise
Biceps	standing curl	curl chin-up	compound curl bicep curl omni curl
Triceps	tricep extension with dumbbells	press down on lat machine	compound tricep tricep extension omni tricep
Forearms	wrist curl	wrist curl	wrist curl on multi exercise
Abdominals/obliques	sit-up side bend with dumbbells	sit-up leg raise	abdominal curl leg raise on multi exercise
Neck	neck bridge (dangerous)	neck harness	4-way neck rotary neck neck and shoulder

5.0 All workouts should begin with the largest muscle groups and proceed down to the smallest.

Sub-principle 5.1 Greater overall strength will result if the largest muscular structures of the body are worked first.

Two reasons are primarily responsible for this sub-principle. (1) When a muscle grows in response to exercise, the entire muscular structures of the body grows to a lesser degree—even muscles that have not been exercised. Thus, the larger the muscle that is growing—or the greater the degree of growth—the greater this overall effect will be. (2) It is almost impossible to reach the required condition of momentary muscular exhaustion in a large muscle if the smaller muscle groups that serve as a link between the resistance and the large muscle groups have been previously exhausted. As a result, it is important to work the largest muscles first—while the system is still capable of working with the desired intensity.

Sub-principle 5.2 Faster rates of growth will result if growth is proportionate.

It is very common for young athletes on a strength training program to ignore the development of their legs entirely, while concentrating on their arms and muscles of the torso. On such a program, the arms will grow to a point, but then additional growth will not occur—or at least not until heavy exercises for the legs are added to the training program. Apparently having reached a maximum permissible degree of disproportionate development, the body will not permit additional arm growth until the legs are also increased in size. Therefore, for the best results from exercise, it is essential that your training program be well rounded—that some form of exercise be included for each of the major muscle masses of your body.

Implications. For best results, the order of exercise should be as follows:

- Hips and lower back
- Legs
    quadriceps
    hamstrings
    calves
- Torso
    back
    shoulders
    chest
- Arms
    triceps
    biceps
    forearms
- Abdominals
- Neck

The hips and legs have the greatest potential for developing strength and muscle mass, so they should be exercised first.

The next body segment to be exercised should be the torso. Generally speaking, when exercising the torso muscles, you should alternate a pressing movement with a pulling movement. By alternating a pressing exercise with a pulling exercise, you will allow the opposing muscles time to recover before performing another exercise.

Always work your arms after the larger and stronger muscles of the torso. To fatigue the smaller and weaker muscle groups of the arms and then perform a torso exercise would provide little benefit for the torso muscles.

When exercising the upper arm muscles (biceps or triceps), you must perform either a pulling or pressing movement. Therefore if the last exercise performed for the torso is a pressing movement (whch involves the triceps) the first exercise for the arms should be a pulling or curling movment (for the biceps), or vice versa.

The forearms should be worked after the biceps and triceps. The reason here is that your grip strength (forearm flexors) is needed to assist in the performance of the other upper body and arm exercies.

Since the abdominal muscles are used in most exercises to stabilize the rib cage and abdominal wall, these muscles should be worked after the arms. To perform high-intensity exercise for the abdominals at an earlier time in your routine would make it difficult to exert a maximum effort on an exercise to follow in which the abdominals act as stabilizers.

You should always work your neck muscles last. Why? Because if these muscles are fatigued first, you'll have a hard time performing an exercise that depends on the support of the head by the neck muscles.

Applying the above guidelines to conventional equipment or Nautilus machines, a basic workout might look as follows:

Conventional Equipment
- Squat (barbell)
- Stiff-legged deadlift (barbell)
- Leg press (leg press machine)
- Bent-armed pullover (barbell or dumbbells)
- Standing press (barbell)
- Chin-up, palms-up grip (horizontal bar)
- Shoulder shrug (dumbbells or barbell)
- Bench press (barbell)
- Standing curl (barbell)
- Dip (parallel bars)
- Sit-up (knees bent)
- Neck harness

Nautilus Machines
- Hip and Back
- Leg Extension
- Leg Press
- Leg Curl
- Pullover
- Double Shoulder
- Neck and Shoulder
- Double Chest
- Bicep/Tricep
- Ab/Ad Machine
- Abdominal Machine
- 4-Way Neck

6.0 Increases in strength are best produced by very brief and infrequent training.

Sub-principle 6.1 High-intensity training must be very brief. It is impossible to have both high-intensity exercise and a large amount of exercise.

In some fashion that is not yet understood, high-intensity work has an effect on the entire system that can be either good or bad, an effect that seldom if ever occurs as a result of low-intensity work. If high-intensity work is followed by an adequate period of rest, then muscular growth and an increase in strength will occur.

So, high intensity work is required for growth stimulation, but it must not be overdone.

Many athletes make the mistake of performing far too much exercise; too many different exercises, too many sets, too many workouts within a given period of time. When an excess amount of exercise is performed, total recovery between workouts becomes impossible; and high-intensity training then becomes equally impossible.

You can have one or the other, but not both. You can perform high-intensity exercise on a brief and infrequent basis with good results. Or you can perform long and frequent low-intensity workouts with very poor results. But you cannot perform long and frequent workouts involving a high-intensity of work. Attempting to do so will produce rapid and large-scale losses in both muscular mass and strength. In addition, it may result in total collapse.

Sub-principle 6.2 Seldom perform more than one set of any exercise in the same training session.

Sub-principle 6.3 A well-supervised, properly conducted, strength-training session should not exceed 30 minutes.

When the requirements for a productive style of high-intensity exercise are understood, it then becomes possible to select the best exercise for a particular purpose. In most cases, not more than 12 different exercises (4-6 for the lower body and 6-8 for the upper body) should be performed in any one training session. If you are "pushed" to an all-out effort in each of the 12 exercises, you will not want to do more than one set of each exercise. In fact, your body will literally "not be able to stand" more than one set.

A set of 10 repetitions performed in proper form (2 seconds on the lifting and 4 seconds on the lowering) should take around one minute to complete. Allowing about one minute between exercises, then most athletes should be able to complete 12 exercises in under 25 minutes. Actually, as the athletes work themselves into better shape, the time between exercises should be reduced. It is entirely possible for a well-conditioned athlete to go through an entire workout (12 exercises) in less than 15 minutes. A workout performed in this fashion not only develops muscular size and strength, but also a high dgree of cardio-respiratory endurance.

Sub-principle 6.4 There should be at least 48 hours rest between high-intensity workouts, but not more than 96 hours.

High-intensity exercise causes a complex chemical reaction to take place inside a muscle. If given time, the body will compensate by causing certain muscle cells to get bigger and stronger. So, high-intensity exercise is necessary in order to stimulate muscular growth; but it is not the only requirement: the stimulated muscle must be **permitted** to grow.

Research has shown that there should be approximately 48 hours between workouts. In some cases, where extremely strong athletes are training, longer periods of time (72 to 96 hours) are required. On the other hand, however, high levels of muscular size and strength start to decrease (atrophy) after about 96 hours of normal activity. So, rest between workouts is important, but not too much rest.

An every-other-day, three times per week exercise program, also seems to provide the body with the needed irregularity of training. The human body quickly grows accustomed to almost any sort of activity—and once having adapted to such activity, then no amount of practice of the same activity will provide growth stimulation. Thus it is important to provide many forms of variation in training. Variation can occur in several different ways: (1) weight and repetitions should be varied for each workout, (2) the exercises can be occasionally changed or alternated or performed in a slightly different sequence, and (3); the training days can be varied. For example, a first workout is performed on Monday, then two days later a second workout is performed on Wednesday, then two days later a third workout is performed on Friday. Thus, on Sunday, the system is expecting and is prepared for a fourth workout, but it does not come. Instead, it comes a day later, on Monday of the next week—when the body is neither expecting it nor prepared for it. This schedule of training prevents the body from falling into a "rut"—since the system is never quite able to adjust to this irregularity of training, and great growth stimulation will be produced as a direct result.

Sub-principle 6.5 An advanced trainee does not need more exercise than a beginner; he needs harder exercise and in most cases less exercise.

Beginning trainees usually show good strength gains on most types of exercise programs, even though they may perform several sets of more than 12 exercises in each training session. They are able to make this progress (at least for a while) because they are simply not strong enough to use all of their recovery ability. As they get stronger, however, they do use up all of their recovery ability—and further growth stops. The stronger the athlete becomes, the greater resistance he handles, and the greater inroads he makes into his overall recovery ability. Therefore, the advanced trainee must reduce his overall exercises (e.g., from 12 to 10) and only train in the high-intensity fashion twice a week. On Monday he might train hard, on Wednesday medium, and on Friday hard. The Wednesday workout would not stimulate growth (the workout would actually keep his muscles from atrophying), it would permit growth by not making significant inroads into the athlete's recovery ability.

Implications. During the off season, all athletes should strength train three times a week. Since most athletes interested in strength training are at a beginning or intermediate level, they should make good progress on three, high-intensity workouts a week. If their progress slows down, they should reduce the high-intensity workouts to two a week, and slightly reduce their total number of exercises. **Never** should the stronger, more advanced trainees perform multiple sets or more than 12 different exercises in any one training session.

Other conditioning drills, especially those performed in a high-intensity fashion (wrestling, sprinting, agility drills, etc.) should be kept at a minimum. Remember, you must have adequtae time (at least two days) to recover from high-intensity work.

During the season, the players need at least one high-intensity workout a week to keep the strength they have developed during the off season. Many athletes, in fact, actually increase their strength during the season by continuing to train hard twice a week. For example, they work out hard the day after a game, and take a second high-intensity workout three days later.

Over a six-month period of time, most trainees should see strength increases of from 50-100% in all the recommended exercises. How much will this added strength improve your athletic ability? Obviously, the answer will vary from athlete to athlete depending on age, prior ability, overall potential, motivation, and many other factors. But in all cases, there will be a measurable degree of improvement and this improvement will produce a level of performance that would not have been reached without proper strength training.

And what degree of protection from injury will be provided by proper strength training? Again the answer will vary; since many complex factors are involved. It should be apparent, however, that a strong limb is far less likely to be injured than a weak one, and it is well established that strength training increases not only the size and strength of muscles, but the connective tissues and even the bones.

In conclusion, the greatest benefits of strength training occur when the exercises are performed in the **proper** manner. The following rules summarize the principles that should be used in organizing a sound strength training program.

1. Select exercises that involve large muscle groups throughout a great range of movement.

2. Stress correct form; avoid fast, jerky movements.

3. Raise the weight to the count of two—lower the weight slowly and evenly while counting to four and repeat.

4. Perform only one set of 8 to 12 repetitions in all exercises.

5. Continue each exercise until no additional repetitions are possible.

6. Attempt to increase repetitions or weight whenever possible.

7. Work the largest muscles first.

8. An entire workout should include a maximum of 12 different exercises.

9. Train no more than three times a week.

10. For best results, you should be supervised and pushed throughout, every workout.

STRENGTH TRAINING—use it properly and you've got everything to gain and nothing to lose.

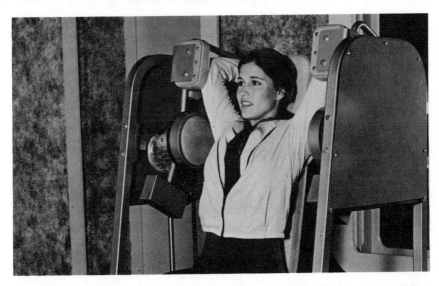

Increases in strength are best produced by very brief and infrequent training.

Bibliography

Allman, Fred L. "Prevention of Sports Injuries" *Athletic Journal* 56:74, March, 1976.

Astrand, Per-Olaf, and Rodahl, Kaare. *Textbook of Work Physiology.* New York: McGraw-Hill, 1970.

Cratty, Bryant J. *Movement Behavior and Motor Learning.* Philadelphia: Lea and Febiger, 1967.

Darden, Ellington. "What Research Says About Positive and Negative Work." *Scholastic Coach* 45:6,7, October, 1975.

DeLorme, T. L., and Watkins, A. L. "Techniques of Progressive Resistance Exercise." *Archives of Physical and Medical Rehabilitation* 29:263-273, 1948.

Goldberg, Alfred L., and others. "Mechanism of Work-Induced Hypertrophy of Skeletal Muscle." *Medicine and Science in Sports* 7:185-198, 1975.

Jokl, Ernst. "Physique and Performance." *American Corrective Therapy Journal* 27:99-114, 1973.

Jones, Arthur. "High Intensity Strength Training." *Scholastic Coach* 42:46, 47, 117, 118, May, 1973.

Jones, Arthur. *Nautilus Training Principles,* Bulletins #1 and #2. DeLand, Florida: Nautilus Sports/Medical Industries, 1970.

Komi, P. V., and Buskirk, E. R. "Effect of Eccentric and Concentric Muscle Conditioning on Tension and Electrical Activity of Human Muscle." *Ergonomics* 15:417-434, 1972.

Lamb, Lawrence E. "Exercise, Muscles." *The Health Letter* 1:#9, 1973.

Larson, Leonard A. *Fitness, Health, and Work Capacity.* New York: MacMillan, 1974.

Peterson, James A. "Total Conditioning: A Case Study." *Athletic Journal* 56:40-55, September, 1975.

Sandow, A. "Excitation-Contraction Coupling in Skeletal Muscle." *Pharmacology Review* 17:265, 1965.

22
Muscle: Structure, Function, and Control

By Michael D. Wolf, Ph.D.
Research Coordinator
Nautilus Sports/Medical Industries, Inc.

Fast twitch. Slow twitch. Red muscle. White muscle. Chances are you've run into one or more of these terms in your travels, and not having a degree in muscle biochemistry, wondered what they meant to you as a coach, trainer, or athlete. The following is an overview of the structure, function, and control of human muscle, always keeping in mind that such knowledge is going to be applied to training and sport.

Q. HOW DOES MUSCLE CONTRACT?

A. Human muscle is, somewhat surprisingly to the non-scientist, over 70% water. Approximately 22% of muscle tissue is protein. Of this latter percentage, the majority is accounted for by millions of strands of a thin filament protein called **actin** and a thick filament protein called **myosin.** Given the presence of calcium, magnesium, and two other proteins called **troponin** and **tropomyosin**, these two filament proteins can contract and move your limbs with great force and great velocity.

The fuel for muscular contraction is a chemical compound called **adenosine triphosphate**, or ATP. When one of the three phosphates is broken off ATP to form ADP, or **adenosine diphosphate**, energy is released into the muscular environment (Figure 1). When actin binds to myosin in the presence of calcium, the energy released from ATP breakdown is used to **pull the actin filaments along the myosin filaments.** More specifically, a bridge forms between actin and myosin. Energy from ATP breakdown is used to shorten the **actomyosin cross-bridge**, which shortens the muscle.

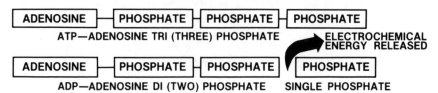

Figure 1 **One phosphate group is broken off ATP to form ADP.
In the process, energy is released.**

Figure 2 shows a simplified unit of muscle called a **sarcomere**. One long strand of many thousands of sarcomeres is called a **myofibril** (Figure 3). Many myofibrils bundled together form one **muscle fiber**. Given the proper input from the nervous system, innervated (switched-on) sarcomeres will contract, and the muscle as a whole will shorten (Figure 4). The process was detailed and named the "Sliding Filament Theory" more than 20 years ago by noted British physiologist H.E. Huxley. Huxley has been internationally honored for his since-proven theory, and is presently Deputy Director of the Molecular Biology Laboratory at Cambridge University in England.

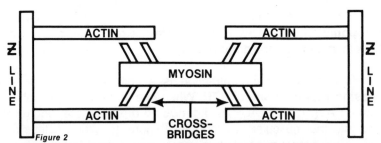

Figure 2

Closeup of one sarcomere. Eight cross-bridges are shown extending from myosin to actin. Given energy from ATP breakdown, these cross-bridges attach to the actin filaments, shorten and telescope the entire Z-line filament units over the myosin filament.

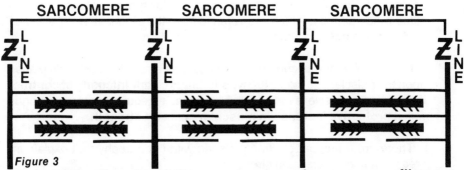

Figure 3
A schematic diagram of three sarcomeres from one myofilament.
Many thousands of sarcomeres form just one myofilament.
Refer to figure 2 for explanation.

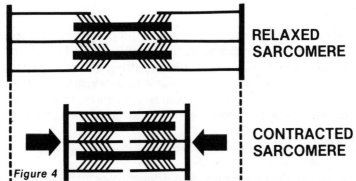

RELAXED
SARCOMERE

CONTRACTED
SARCOMERE

Figure 4
When cross-bridges pull Z-lines together, sarcomere length
decreases, but neither actin nor myosin filaments shorten.

Q. HOW DOES MUSCLE GROW?

A. The technical term for muscular growth is **hypertrophy**. Its inverse, called **atrophy**, refers to the breakdown of muscle tissue from disuse. The process of atrophy involves metabolic breakdown of muscle into its constituent compounds, which are removed via the bloodstream. Atrophied muscle **does not** turn into fat.

Hypertrophy, or muscular growth, occurs as a result of demands placed upon the muscle. The signal for hypertrophy is clearly **intensity of contraction**. When a muscle is faced with high intensity requirements, it responds with a **protective increase in muscular size and strength**.

There are a number of changes seen with hypertrophy that explain increased muscular size and strength:
- The actin and particularly the myosin protein filaments increase in size.
- The number of myofibrils (lengths of actin/myosin units, or "sarcomeres") increases.
- The number of blood capillaries within the fiber may increase.
- The amount and strength of connective tissue within the muscle may increase.
- The number of muscle fibers (which consist of many myofibrils) may increase.

There is heavy scientific debate over the occurrence of this last phenomenon, which is called **hyperplasia.** While a small number of studies on rats and cats have shown hyperplasia, or **fiber splitting** with increased muscular size, most researchers have not been able to demonstrate it. As of 1981, there is no evidence that the number of muscle fibers increases in humans when muscular size and strength are increased through weight training.

Q. ARE THERE DIFFERENT TYPES OF MUSCLE?

A. In the middle 1970's there was some debate over just how many types of muscle could be found in humans. International consensus has since firmly established a four-category classification of human muscle. The only confusion that exists at present is in the naming of the categories. There is no disagreement in international circles over the fact that four distinct types of muscle fiber exist in man, however. Table 1 presents the three major classification schemes for the four types of human muscle fiber.

The four fiber types differ on a great number of characteristics. The three most important are force of contraction, speed of contraction, and endurance.

Table 1

THREE CLASSIFICATION SCHEMES

THE FOUR FIBER TYPES		
—I—	—SO— SLOW, OXIDATIVE	—S— SLOW,
—II A —	—FO— FAST, OXIDATIVE	—FR— FAST, FATIGUE RESISTANT
—II AB —	-FOG- FAST, OXIDATIVE PLUS GLYCOLYTIC	—FI— FAST, INTERMEDIATE FATIGUEABILITY
—II B —	—FG— FAST, GLYCOLYTIC	—FF— FAST, FATIGUEABLE

Referring back to Table 1, note that three of the four fiber types are characterized as fast. Only the type I fibers are slow in contraction speed. They were once called the red, or slow-twitch fibers, but the "red-white" and "slow-twitch, fast twitch" classification systems are no longer used by physiologists. The word "oxidative" (Table 1) refers to the ability of the muscle tissue to use oxygen for long periods of time to synthesize and make use of ATP.

The three fast fibers differ from each other most in endurance. The IIa fibers have a high endurnce factor despite being fast and powerful. They do not have the long-term endurance of the slow, type I fibers, however. The IIb fibers are the powerful sprint fibers that fatigue most quickly. The term "glycolytic" refers to the ability of type II fibers to function well, but for short periods of time, without oxygen. Between the IIa and IIb fibers in endurance ability lie the IIab fibers. Though the issue is far more complicated than the following examples will suggest, for now picture the type I fibers as the marathon runner's "best friend" and the type IIb fibers as the sprinter's "best friend."

Q. DOES EVERYONE HAVE ALL FOUR KINDS OF MUSCLE?

A. Generally speaking, all four muscle fiber types can be seen in the body, but their percentages vary greatly from muscle to muscle. For example, the gastrocnemius (the most prominent part of the calf) can be almost wholly type II, while the soleus, lying below the gastrocnemius, can be almost wholly type I. Most of our muscles, however, contain a mix of all four fiber types.

The percentage of each fiber type seen in a muscle appears to be genetically fixed. Research has shown fairly conclusively that training has a small or negligible effect on the fiber composition of muscle. What that means is this: if you were born with deltoids and triceps that are largely composed of IIb fibers, you have much greater potential in athletic events such as the shotput than if those muscles were type I. Conversely, if your hamstrings and quadriceps are largely type I you have an enhanced potential for success at distance running. To a great extent, elite athletes are born and not made.

Q. HOW DOES THE BRAIN CALL UPON AND USE MUSCLE?

A. It was once thought that the thin, gray **motor cortex**, sitting on top of the brain, was in complete control of movement. Plans were made, commands issued downward, and the muscle snapped into action. It is now

238

known that the motor cortex is the **last** brain structure to act before movement, rather than the **first**. Plans appear to be made in the **frontal cortex**, movements initiated and coordinated in the **basal ganglia** and **cerebellum** then relayed through the thalamus, and final commands directed from **motor cortex** downward into the **spinal cord.** It is also known that there are a number of spinal pathways that can carry commands from brain centers **other than the motor cortex** directly to the muscle (Figure 5).

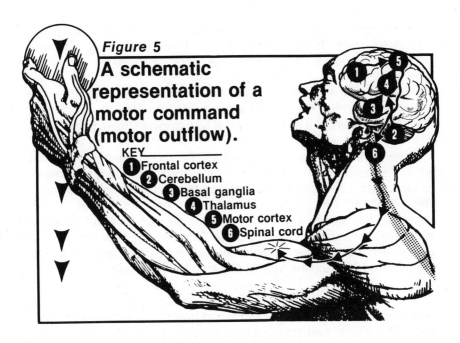

Figure 5

A schematic representation of a motor command (motor outflow).

KEY

1 Frontal cortex
2 Cerebellum
3 Basal ganglia
4 Thalamus
5 Motor cortex
6 Spinal cord

When a message from any of the brain centers, called **supraspinal** (above the spine) **centers**, reaches the spinal cord, it is transmitted to the muscle via the **motorneuron**. These structures are simply nerves that carry motor commands. The number of muscle fibers that one motorneuron can control varies from as little as one to as many as several hundred. One motorneuron, and **all** the muscle fibers it controls, is called a **motor unit**. When a motorneuron turns on its muscle fibers, they must contract fully in one burst. The principle that an individual muscle fiber is either completely "on" or completely "off" is called the **all-or-none law.**

The natural question that the all-or-none law raises is: "How can we get different forces of contraction, or **graded contraction**, if muscle fibers are either on or off?" The answer is that the brain only calls on the number and types of muscle fibers that it needs. When the need for more force arises, the brain has a number of options. One of these is to simply ask or **recruit** more all-or-none fibers. The other is to stimulate the fibers it **has already called on**, or **recruited**, more rapidly. There is a sizeable debate going on concerning how much the brain relies on "more fibers" versus "faster stimulation" when more force is needed.

To summarize thus far, the brain estimates the number and type of fibers it needs for a task, then recruits them in an all-or-none fashion. If these fibers are not enough, the brain will do one of several things:

- Stimulate the already-on fibers more rapidly (frequency)
- Ask for more of the same fibers to join in (recruitment)
- Ask for fibers of a **more powerful** type to join in (recruitment)

Hidden in this last sentence is perhaps the most important point in this whole discussion. There is a wealth of evidence that in nearly all human endeavors the brain follows the **size principle of recruitment**. This principle states that recruitment order is based upon increasing size of motorneurons. Most simply, small motorneurons are called upon first, and the largest motorneurons are recruited last. Since muscle fiber size correlates closely with the size order of motorneurons, the type I fibers (the smallest) are recruited first, and the type IIb (the largest) are recruited last.

Nearly all evidence suggests that in humans it is the **intensity or force requirements** that determine which and how many muscle fibers will be used. There is no evidence that the speed of contraction determines fiber recruitment. In other words, the brain recruits muscle based on how much force the muscle must create, and not on how fast it must contract. The simple explanation for this is that so-called "slow-twitch" or type I fibers are fully capable of moving the limbs at extreme velocities (greater than 1000 degrees per second) **if the force requirements are low**. Training rapidly but with low intensity **cannot** prepare the muscle for high intensity athletic performance.

For low intensity muscular work, the small type I fibers (the smallest of the four types) will suffice. Once the type I fibers become insufficient for the task, the brain will recruit the next **larger** fiber types or the IIa or IIab fibers. When even the I, IIa, and IIab fibers cannot meet the force requirements the brain will, **as a last resort**, recruit the largest type IIb fibers. All **four** fiber types are working when IIb fibers are recruited. Athletic performance requiring movements of power and speed utilize all four fiber types but are most dependent on the IIb fibers. There is **no** firm evidence in humans that **any movement**, at **any speed,** can cause the brain to **preferentially recruit IIb [formerly "fast-twitch"] fibers**. Such preferential recruitment, the bypassing of I, IIa, and IIab fibers, has been shown in extremely rapid, low force movements in cats, but no researcher has been able to demonstrate it in humans.

Q. WHY THEN DO MANY COACHES AND EQUIPMENT MANUFACTURERS ADVOCATE HIGH SPEED TRAINING?

A. Such training advice can be blamed on a lack of knowledge of basic neuromuscular physiology and a great deal of poorly-conducted research. Most laymen, and unfortunately many exercise researchers, assume that slow-twitch (type I) fibers are only responsible for slow movements. As noted above, the type I fibers may move a limb at extreme speeds **if the load is light**. Once loading assumes the proportions of a 200 pound offensive lineman, type IIa and IIb fibers must also be recruited. Neglect of these neurophysiological principles has been based on several widely-published studies, but none as much as the work by Moffroid and Whipple (1970) in the Journal of The American Physical Therapy Association.

The authors trained one experimental group on isokinetic knee extension at a high intensity and low speed (36 degrees per second). A second experimental group was trained at what the authors **called** a fast speed. Since human limbs may exceed one thousand degrees per second in angular velocity, it is clear that this second group, training at 108 degrees per second, was not training at a high speed. Nevertheless, this latter speed has been accepted by the community as "fast." A third group was tested before and after the six week training period, but was not trained. After the six weeks, the three groups were tested at zero degrees per second (isometrically) and at six speeds from 18 to 108 degrees per second.

Moffroid and Whipple conducted that training at a "fast" speed led to strength gains at all speeds tested while the "slow" group only gained in strength at slow speeds. **This conclusion has been cited literally hundreds of times since 1970 as evidence that training should occur at high speed and low intensity.** The data from Moffroid and Whipple (1970) are presented here exactly as they appeared in print (Table 2), and both of the original peak torque curves (which had appeared separately) are plotted for comparison on one graph (Figure 6).

Table 2

Mean Increases of Peak Torque for Quadriceps

Velocity	Group I Newton Meters	Group II Newton Meters	Group III Newton Meters
	SLOW	FAST	CONTROL
0 rpm	28.6	21.8	14.1
3 rpm	35.4	16.8	3.9
6 rpm	47.1	24.8	8.3
9 rpm	14.5	14.5	8.4
12 rpm	14.1	17.5	6.9
15 rpm	10.8	12.3	4.8
18 rpm	8.4	15.6	2.0

from: M. MOFFROID & R WHIPPLE. SPECIFICITY OF SPEED AND EXERCISE. JOURNAL OF THE AMERICAN PHYSICAL THERAPY ASSOCIATION Volume 50 : 1699, 1970.

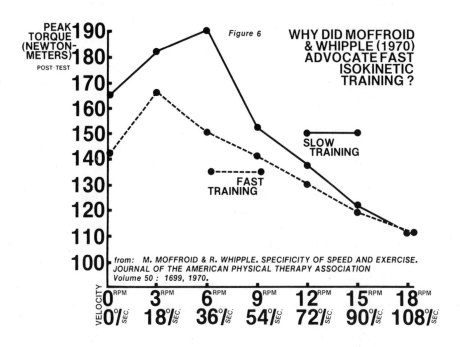

The **data absolutely do not support the authors' conclusions.** If for no other reason, the conclusions are valueless because the authors violated a basic principle of statistical analysis: when pre-tests indicated that one group had higher mean peak torques at all speeds, analysis of **post-test** data should have employed a technique known as "analysis of covariance." This tool **statistically equates** the two groups on **pre-test** data so that **post-test** results can be compared fairly. Given the initial differences found by Moffroid and Whipple, their use of analysis of variance, and not **co**variance, prevents consideration of any of their conclusions.

Despite this failure, the results can be reinspected. A close analysis of the data reveals that the **only statistically significant differences** between groups were at two lower speeds, where the slow group showed nearly **twice** the gains of the fast group (Table 2). In the case where fast outgained slow, the differences were not only of much smaller magnitude, but **were not statistically significant**. In layman's terms, failure to reach significance means only one thing: the differences **cannot be attributed to training method.**

Moffroid and Whipple, even in the light of the above, stated that the fast group increased in strength at all speeds while the slow group increased only at slow speeds. It should be obvious that such conclusions were incorrect and totally unsupported by the data. In fact, according to the principles of statistics and experimental design, all their analyses were incorrect. It is sad that so many have cited this study as evidence that training should occur at fast speeds.

Q. WHAT THEN IS THE MOST EFFECTIVE WAY TO STRENGTHEN MUSCLE?

A. There is solid evidence that slow, high intensity training causes the brain to recruit the I, IIa, and IIb fibers in an orderly fashion. There is no evidence that fast, low intensity training preferentially works the IIb fibers. Remember that type I fibers are perfectly capable of moving limbs at extremely rapid speeds (over 1000 degrees per second) if the force requirements are low. Training at high intensity appears to be the **only way** to maximally use the IIb fibers.

A further problem with high speed training is that the only way to move a heavy load rapidly is to "explode" into it. Two very definite things occur with explosive movement, and both of them are unacceptable and potentially destructive.

In terms of safety, the forces created in such a movement can easily exceed the structural integrity of muscle, connective and bone tissue. Explosive training is, sooner or later, a sure ticket to the orthopedic surgeon's office.

Furthermore, when a barbell or load is moved explosively, the weight is given sufficient momentum to work under its own power. Such movement is called **ballistic**. Note on the oscilloscope tracing in Figure 7 that the load on the muscles in an explosive, 60 pound barbell military press is **below** 60 pounds for almost half the movement! Quite obviously, if the load on the muscle significantly decreases below 60 pounds, the muscle is **not being trained**. Given the inherent dangers and the ineffective loading of the musculature, one wonders why any athlete would be coached to train explosively.

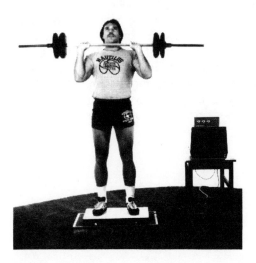

Figure 7. A force plate is a measuring device that is used to measure changes in force. Pictured above is a subject standing on a force plate that is connected to an oscilloscope. As the subject performs an overhead press, the forces are recorded. If the movement is performed in a smooth, steady manner, the signal on the screen will travel across the scope in a relatively straight line fashion. If the barbell is pressed in a fast, explosive style, the signal will move wildly up and down the scope, thereby accurately indicating the changing levels of force imposed upon the subject.

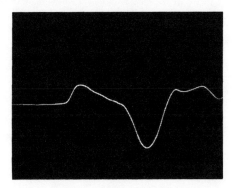

An actual tracing of the changing forces involved in rapid exercise is shown in this photo. Notice the peaks and drops in the tracing. A 60-pound barbell—if suddenly jerked or thrown—can exert a force of several hundred pounds, or can exert a force that literally measures below zero! Such rapid exercise is not only unproductive as far as strength training is concerned, but is also very dangerous to the joints, muscles, and connective tissues.

In conclusion, the great weight of evidence suggests that the most effective way to train human muscle is to work it at great intensity and slow speed. Research and experience from major projects at Colorado State University and The United States Military Academy at West Point, and ongoing work at Nautilus headquarters in Lake Helen, Florida, support the concept that optimal strength training requires as little as one set of eight to twelve repetitions taken to momentary muscular failure. Many questions remain, but their answers are being actively pursued.

23
Nautilus Training

By John P. Donati
Marketing Coordinator
Nautilus Sports/Medical Industries, Inc.

Nautilus is, first and foremost, a concept. A Nautilus machine is a manifestation of both the Nautilus concept and what research has shown to be the most efficient vehicle for implementing that concept.

Conventional exercises work only part of a muscle. A Nautilus machine, however, works all of a muscle. With conventional exercises, there are limitations to the results, which can be achieved because of design limitations in the tools themselves. With Nautilus, the results are limited only by the God-given potential of the individual who is exercising.

Function dictates design. And Nautilus is the only equipment that considers the function of the muscle as the primary prerequisite for the design of the machines. The basic concept behind every Nautilus machine is the isolation and exercise of specific muscle groups with correct form and method.

Similar to any tool, a Nautilus machine is only as good as the way it is used. In order to receive maximum benefit from the use of a Nautilus machine, proper form must be followed. This chapter presents quidelines regarding the correct usage of Nautilus equipment.

HIP AND BACK MACHINE

Muscles Involved: Gluteus Maximus

Procedure:

- Lie face up with both legs over the roller pads.

- Grasp the handles lightly and straighten arms. The hip joint should now be aligned with the rotational axis of the cam.

- Fasten the seat belt so that the back may be arched at the completion of the movement. The belt should be snug but not too tight.

- Press the right roller pad toward the floor by fully extending the right leg. Now smoothly extend the left leg to parallel with the right leg. This is the fully contracted position.

- Keeping one leg contracted, allow the other leg to bend slowly toward the chest. This is the stretched position.

- Return to the fully contracted position.

- Pause and repeat with the other leg.

Note: In the contracted position, keep the legs straight and knees together. Toes should remain pointed throughout the movement.

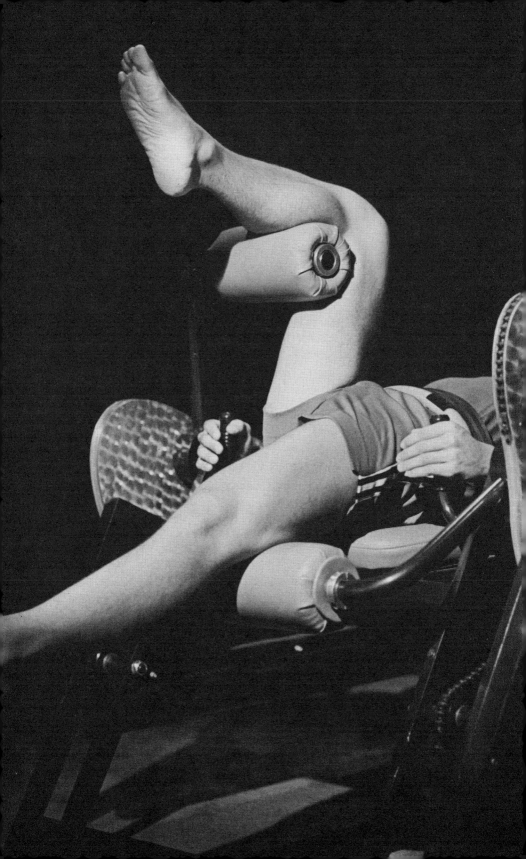

LEG EXTENSION MACHINE

Muscles Involved: Quadriceps

Procedure:

- In the seated position, place the feet behind the roller pads with the knees snugly against the seat pad.

- Pull the seat back forward to touch the lower back.

- Keep the head and shoulders relaxed against the seat back.

- Straighten the legs smoothly to the fully contracted position and pause.

- Slowly lower the resistance and repeat the movement. Do not let the weight rest on the weight stack.

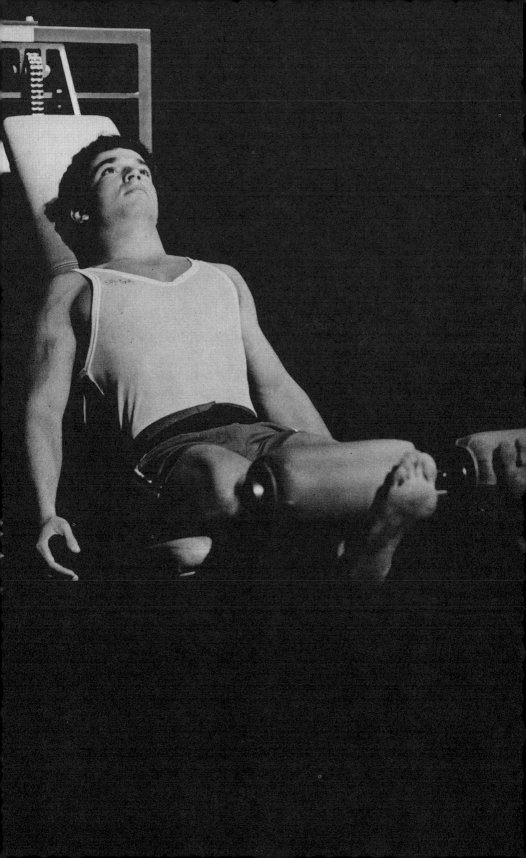

LEG CURL MACHINE

Muscles Involved: Hamstrings

Procedure:

- Lie face down on the machine with the knees just off the edge of the pad.
- Place the feet under the roller pads.
- Lightly grasp the handles.
- Curl the legs, trying to touch the heels to the buttocks.
- When lower legs are perpendicular to the bench, lift the buttocks to relax the quadriceps thus increasing the range of movement in the hamstrings.
- Pause at the point of full muscular contraction.
- Slowly lower the resistance and repeat.

Note: The top of the foot should be flexed toward the knees throughout the movement.

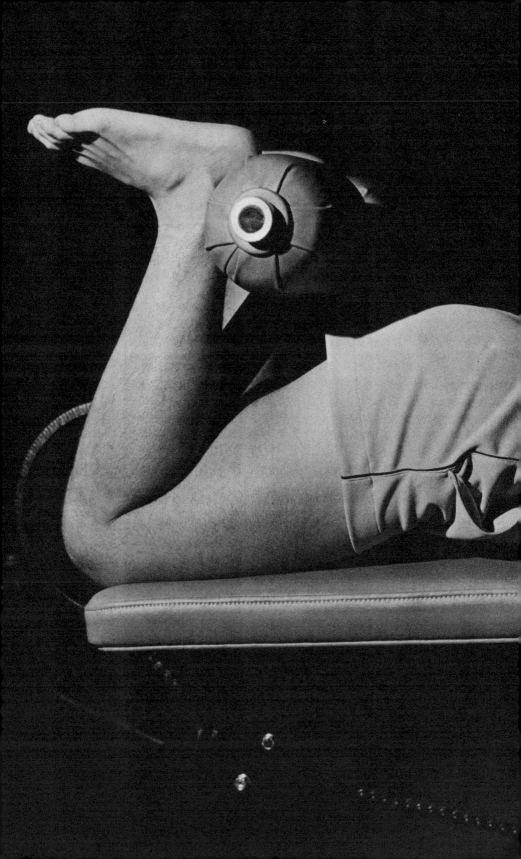

HIP ABDUCTION/ ADDUCTION MACHINE

Hip Abduction
Muscles Involved: Gluteus medius
Procedure:

- Adjust the lever on the right side of the machine until both movement arms are together.

- Move the thigh pads to the outer position.

- Sit in the machine and place the knees and ankles on the movement arms. The outer thighs and knees should be firmly against the resistance pads.

- Keep the head and shoulders relaxed against the seat back.

- Spread the knees and thighs to the widest possible position and pause.

- Return slowly to the starting position and repeat.

Hip Adduction
Muscles Involved: Adductor magnus
Procedure:

- Adjust the lever on the right side of the machine until the movement arms are as wide as comfortably possible.

- Move the thigh pads to the inside position.

- Sit in the machine and place the knees and ankles on the movement arms. The inner thighs and knees should be firmly against the resistance pads.

- Keep the head and shoulders relaxed against the seat back.

- Press the knees and thighs smoothly together and pause.

- Return slowly to the starting position and repeat.

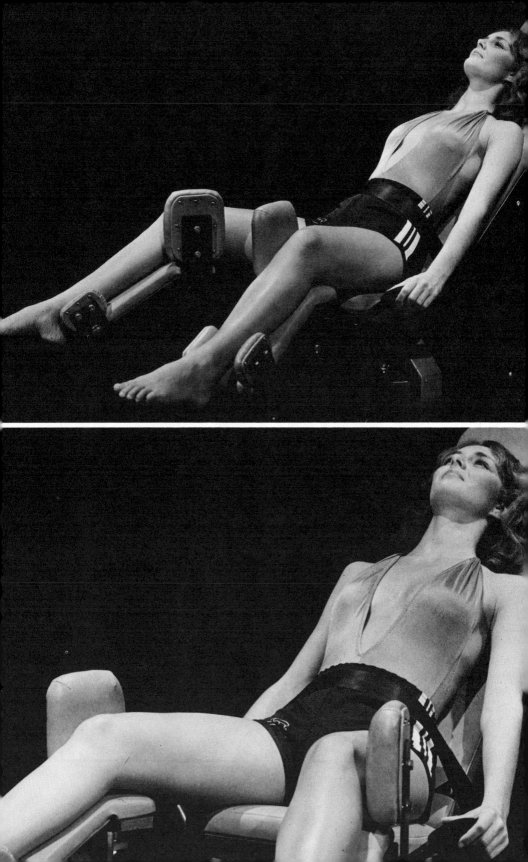

PULLOVER MACHINE

Muscles Involved: Latissimus dorsi

Procedure:

- Adjust the seat so the shoulder joints are in line with the axes of the cams. (The top of the shoulder should be in line with the center of the side pad.)
- Sit erect and fasten the seat belt.
- Press the foot pedal to bring the elbow pads within reach.
- Place the elbows on the pads. The hands should be open and resting on the movement arm.
- Remove the feet from the pedal, allowing the movement arm to rotate as far back as possible. This is the stretched position.
- With the elbows, drive the movement arm around to the mid-section and pause.
- Slowly return to the stretched position and repeat.

Note: Look straight ahead during the movement, keeping the head and torso still. Do not grip or pull with the hands.

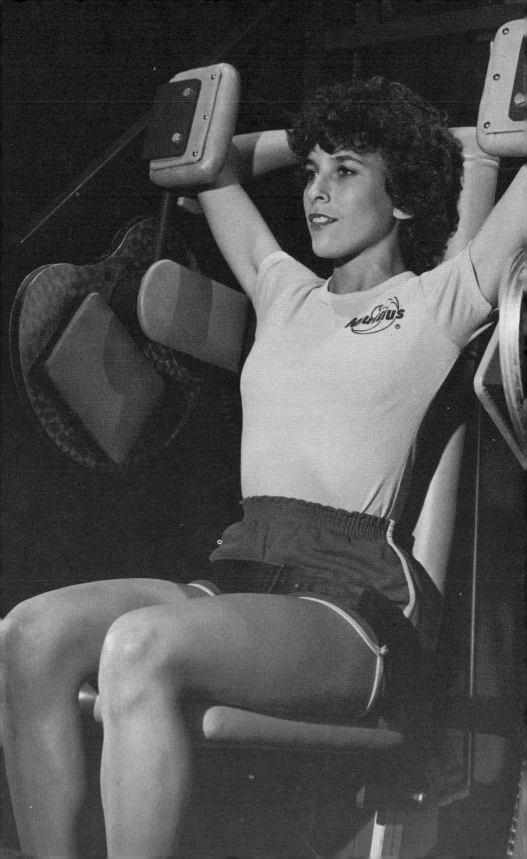

BEHIND NECK MACHINE

Behind Neck
Muscles Involved: Latissimus dorsi
Procedure:

- Adjust the seat so the shoulder joints are in line with the axes of the cams.
- Fasten the seat belt.
- Place the back of the upper arms between the padded movement arms.
- Cross the forearms behind the neck.
- Drive the elbows downward until the forearms are perpendicular to the floor and pause.
- Slowly return the arms to the crossed position behind the neck and repeat.
- After the final repetitions, immediately perform the behind neck pulldown movement.

Note: Be careful not to bring the arms or hands to the front of the body.

Behind Neck Torso Arm
Muscles Involved: Biceps and latissimus dorsi
Procedure:

- Lean forward and grasp the overhead bar with a parallel grip.
- Keeping the elbows back, pull the bar behind the neck and pause.
- Slowly return to the starting position and repeat.

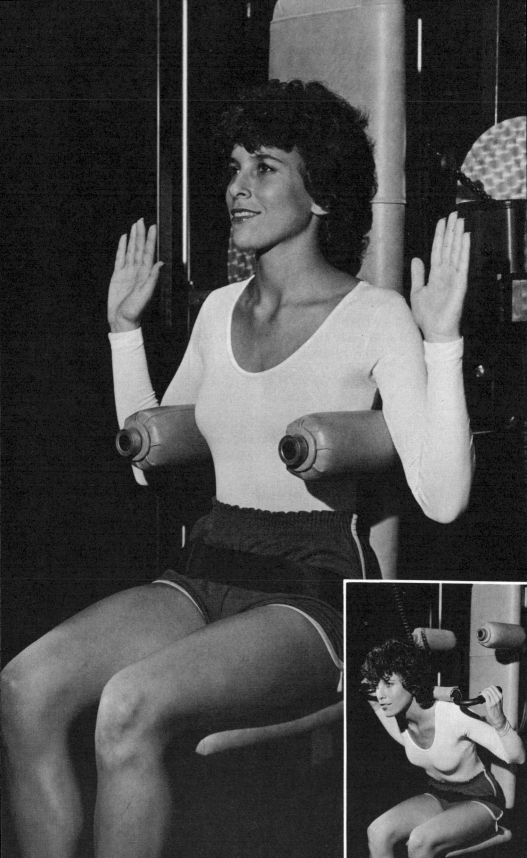

DOUBLE CHEST MACHINE

Double Chest
Muscles Involved: Pectoralis major
Procedure:

- Adjust the seat so that, in the contracted position (elbows together), the shoulders are directly under the axes of the overhead cams. (The elbows should be slightly higher than parallel to the floor.)

- Fasten the seat belt.

- Place the forearms behind and firmly against the movement arm pads and lightly grasp the handles.

- Bring the movement arms together by leading with the elbows and pause.

- Slowly lower the resistance and repeat.

- After the final repetition, immediately perform the decline press movement.

Note: The head and upper body must remain relaxed against the seat back.

Decline Press
Muscles Involved: Pectorals, deltoids and triceps
Procedure:

- Bring the handles into the starting position by pressing the foot pedal.

- Grasp the handles with a parallel grip.

- Press the handles forward. Do not lock the elbows.

- Slowly lower the resistance as far back as possible without distorting the grip. Keep the elbows comfortably away from the body.

- Repeat the movement.

Note: Keep the head and torso erect.

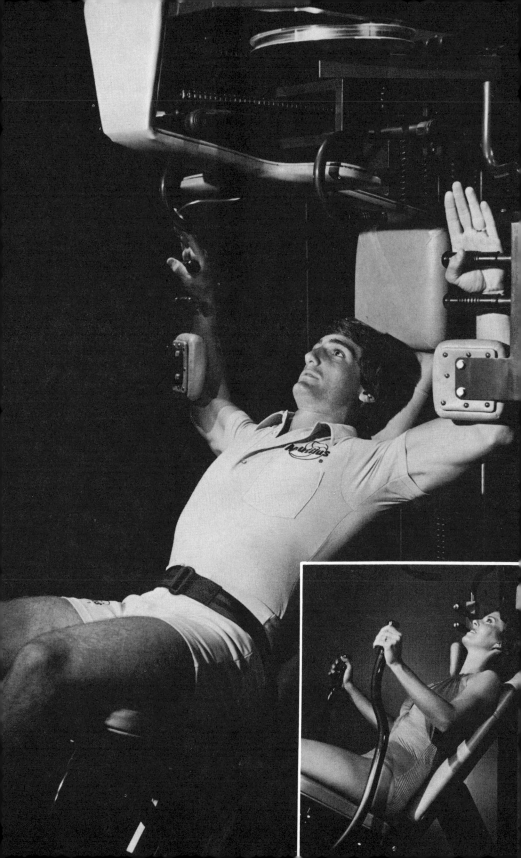

ROWING TORSO MACHINE

Muscles Involved: Posterior deltoids and rhomboids

Procedure:

- Sit with the back toward the weight stack.
- Place the arms between the roller pads. Cross the arms keeping the elbows in the center of the pads with the forearms parallel to the floor.
- Drive the elbows as far back as possible and pause.
- Slowly return to the starting position and repeat.

Note: Do not lean forward.

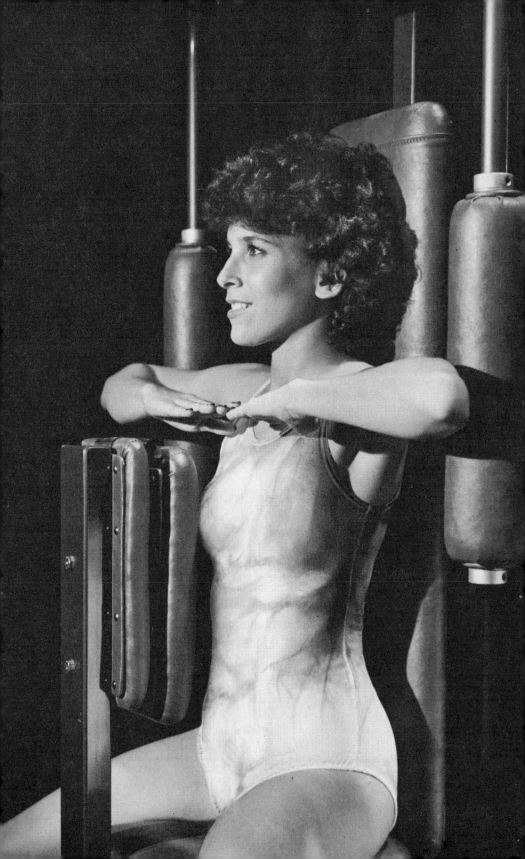

DOUBLE SHOULDER MACHINE

Double Shoulder
Muscles Involved: Deltoids
Procedure:

- Adjust the seat so the shoulder joints are in line with the axes of the cams.
- Fasten the seat belt.
- Lightly grasp the handles.
- Raise both arms until parallel to the floor and pause. Be sure to lead with the elbows.
- Slowly lower the resistance and repeat.
- After the final repetition, immediately perform the overhead press.

Note: The head and shoulders must remain relaxed against the seat back.

Overhead Press
Muscles Involved: Deltoids and
  triceps
Procedure:

- Grasp the handles located above the shoulder.
- Press the handles straight up. Do not lock the elbows.
- Slowly lower the resistance, keeping the elbows wide and repeat.

Note: Do not arch the back. Thighs should be resting on the seat throughout both exercises.

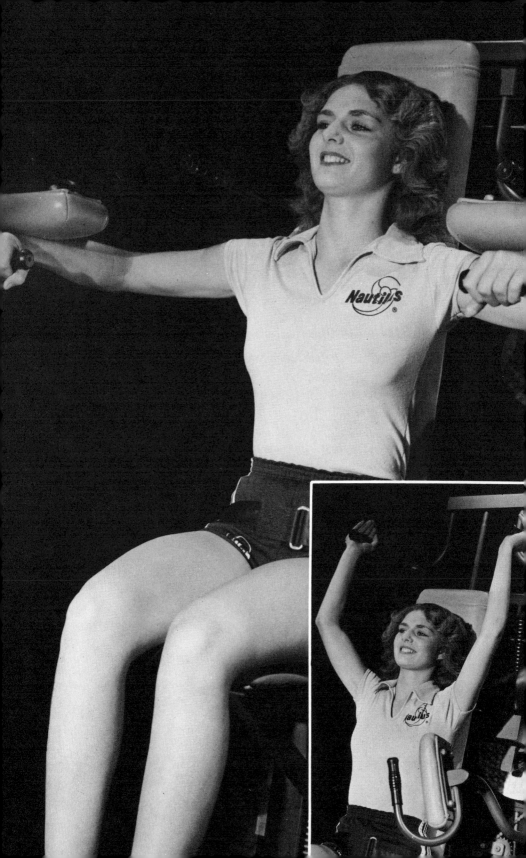

NECK AND SHOULDER MACHINE

Muscles Involved: Trapezius

Procedure:

- While seated, place forearms between the pads.
- Keep the palms open with the fingers pointed toward the floor.
- When sitting erect, weight stack should be elevated. (Seat pads may be required.)
- While extending fingers to the floor, raise the shoulders as high as possible and pause.
- Slowly return to the stretched position and repeat.

Note: Do not lean back or push with the feet.

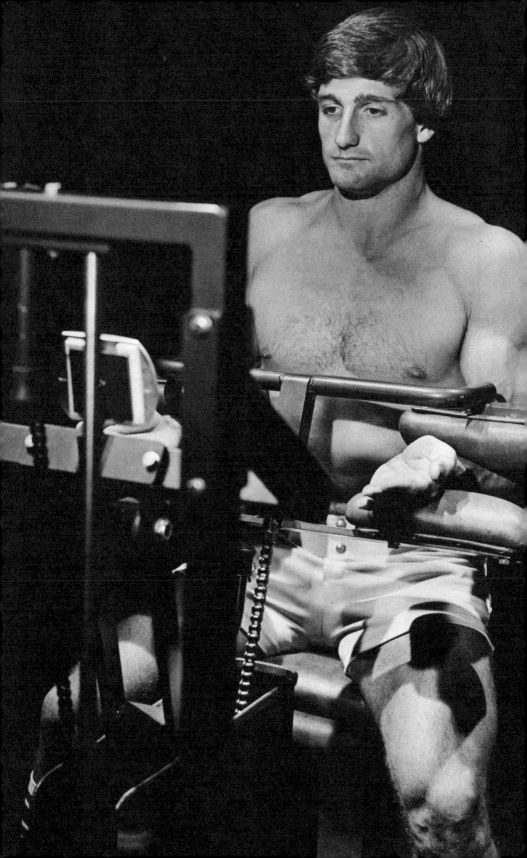

BICEPS CURL MACHINE

Muscles Involved: Biceps

Procedure:

- Place the elbows on the pad and in line with the axes of the cams. (Elbows should be slightly higher than the shoulders.)
- Lightly grasp the handles with the palms up.
- Curl the left movement arm smoothly to the shoulder and pause.
- Slowly return to the starting position and repeat the movement with the right arm.

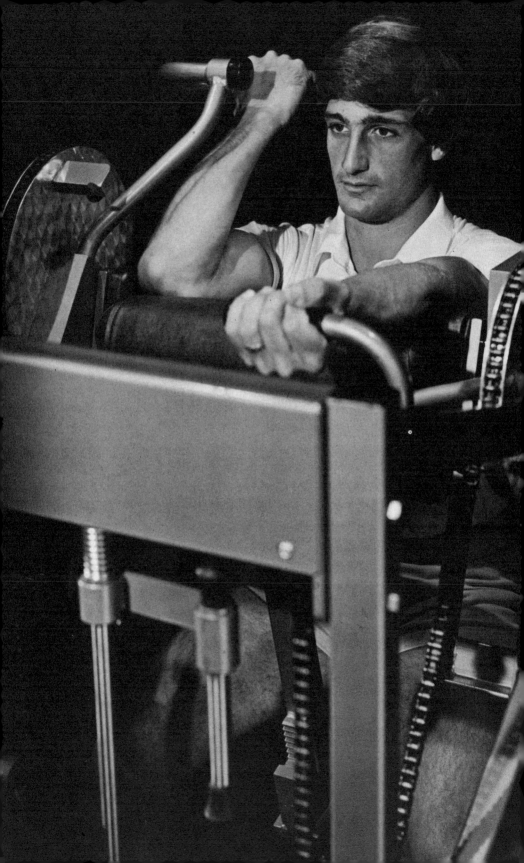

TRICEPS EXTENSION MACHINE

Muscles Involved: Triceps

Procedure:

- Place the elbows on the pad in line with the axes of the cams. (Elbows should be slightly higher than the shoulders.)
- Hands must be placed on the pads in a "karate chop" position.
- Straighten the left arm smoothly to position of full extension and pause. Return to the starting position.
- Repeat with the right arm.

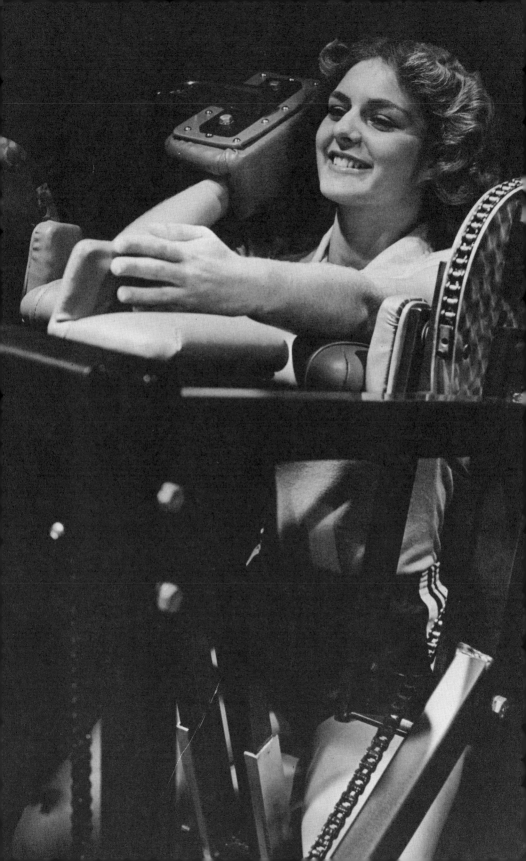

4-WAY NECK MACHINE

Muscles Involved: Sterno-mastoid, splenius, and other neck muscles

Procedure:

ANTERIOR FLEXION

- Face the machine and adjust the seat so the nose is centered between the pads.
- Sit erect and lightly grasp the handles.
- Smoothly move the head toward the chest and pause.
- Slowly return to the starting position and repeat.

POSTERIOR FLEXION

- Place the back of the head in contact with the center of the pads.
- Sit erect and lightly grasp the handles.
- Extend the head as far back as possible and pause.
- Slowly return to the starting position and repeat.

LATERAL CONTRACTION

- Adjust the seat so the left ear is centered between the pads.
- Sit erect and lightly grasp the handles.
- Smoothly move the head toward the left shoulder and pause.
- Keep the shoulders level through the movement.
- Slowly return to the starting position and repeat.

Follow the same procedure for the right side.

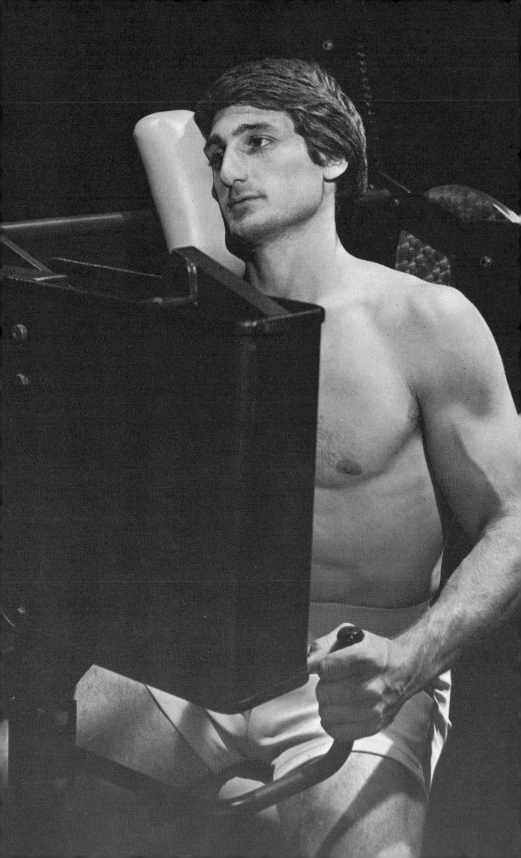

ABDOMINAL MACHINE

Muscles Involved: Rectus Abdominis

Procedure:

- Adjust the seat so the lower part of the sternum is even with the lower edge of the top pad.
- Place the ankles behind the roller pads.
- Spread the legs and sit erect.
- Grasp the handles and keep the elbows high.
- The shoulders and head should remain against the pad.
- Shorten the distance between the rib cage and the navel by contracting the abdominals. Do not pull with the arms or lift up with the legs. Pause in the contracted position.
- Return to the starting position and repeat.

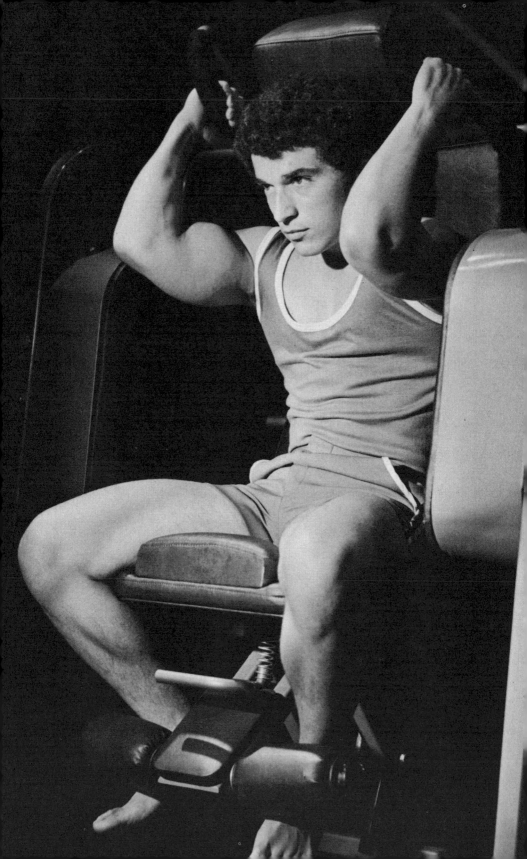

ROTARY TORSO MACHINE

Muscles Involved: Obliques (external and internal) and erector spinea

Procedure:

- Adjust the seat yoke 90 degrees to the right of the weight stack.
- Straddle the seat and restrict lower body movement by crossing the ankles.
- Turn to the right and with forearms resting on the pads lightly grasp the center bar.
- Rotate the torso from the right to the left by pushing with the right palm. Use torso rotators and do not pull with the left arm.
- Pause in the contracted position.
- Head movement should be consistent with the torso movement.
- Return to the starting position and repeat.
- Reverse the seat and the procedures for left to right torso rotation.

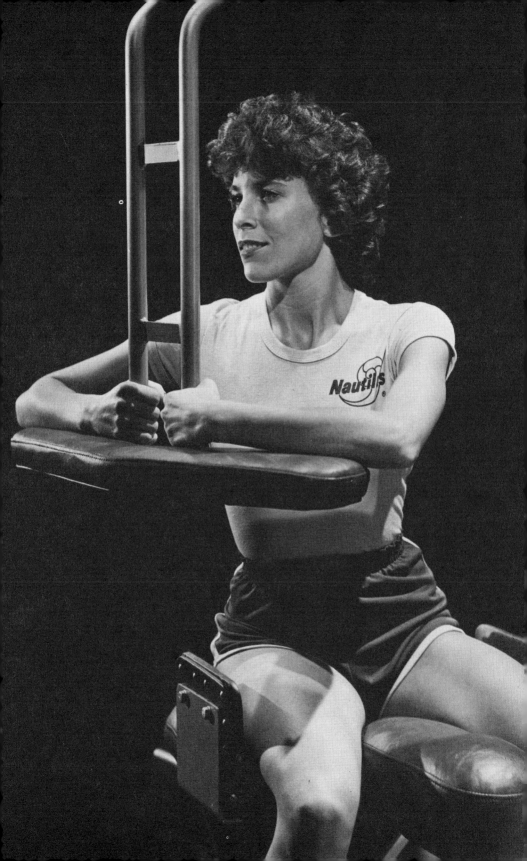

MULTI-EXERCISE MACHINE

Calf Raises
Muscles Involved: Gastrocnemius
Procedure:

- Adjust the belt comfortably above the hips.
- Place the balls of the feet on the first step and the hands on the carriage bar.
- Keep the knees locked throughout the entire movement.
- Raise the heels as high as possible and pause.
- Slowly lower the heels and stretch at the bottom by lifting the toes.
- Repeat.

Wrist Curl
Muscles Involved: Forearm flexors
Procedure:

- Sit on a bench in front of the machine with the toes under the first step.
- Grasp the handles with palms up.
- Rest the forearms against the thighs.
- Slowly curl the wrists upward and pause.
- Slowly lower the resistance and repeat.

Note: Do not move forearms. A palms-down grip may also be used.

Other Exercises for the Multi-Exercise Machine:

Chin-up	Hanging Leg Raise
Parallel Dip	Side Bend
Bent-Over Row	Triceps Extension
Shoulder Shrug	Biceps Curl

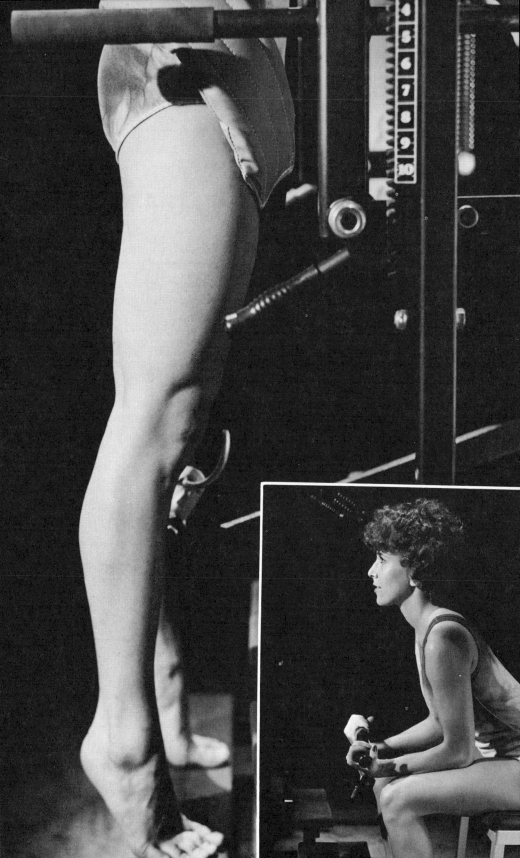

RULES FOR NAUTILUS TRAINING

- Perform one set of 4-6 exercises for the lower body and 6-8 exercises for the upper body. The total number of exercises should not exceed 12.
- Select a resistance that will allow between 8-12 repetitions.
- Continue each exercise to a point of momentary muscular failure.
- When 12 or more repetitions are performed in perfect form, increase the resistance 5 percent the next exercise session.
- Exercise the larger muscle groups first and proceed down to the smaller muscle groups (example: hips, thighs, back, chest, shoulders, arms, neck.)
- Raise the weight on a two count; lower the weight on a four count. When in doubt about the speed of movement, go slower.
- Attempt to increase the number of repetitions or the amount of resistance every workout. But never sacrifice form in an attempt to get "one more rep."
- Train no more than three times per week. Allow at least 48 hours between workouts, but no more than 96 hours.
- Keep accurate records of each workout. Date, resistance, repetitions, and overall workout time should be recorded.
- The entire workout should take from 20 to 30 minutes.

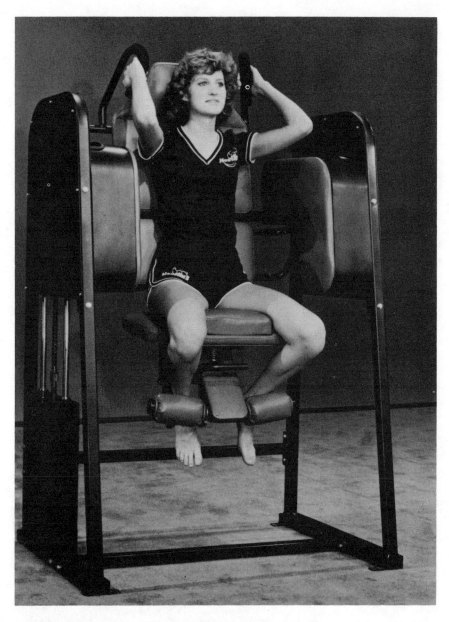

In terms of achieving maximal results in the least amount of time and in the safest way possible, more is definitely not better.

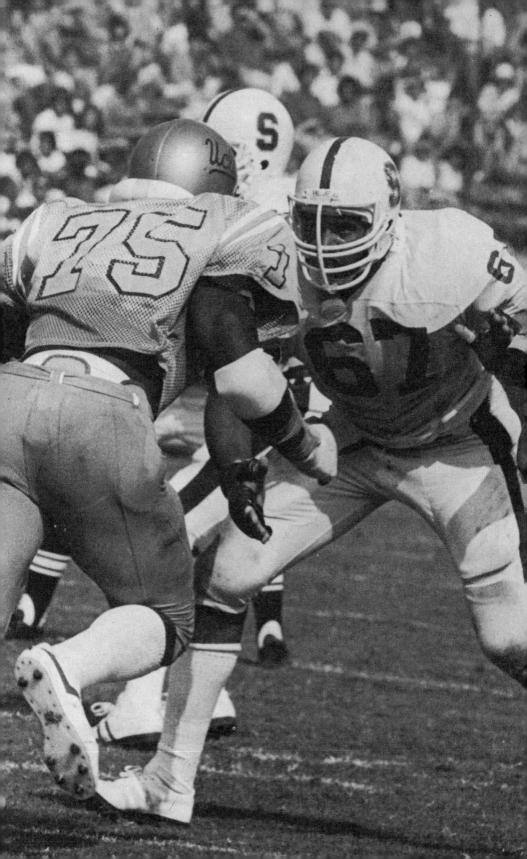

24
STRENGTH TRAINING: PREVENTIVE MEDICINE FOR THE ATHLETE*

By Michael N. Fulton, M.D.
Orthopaedic and Rehabilitation Clinic
Lake Helen, Florida

As in most physical endeavors, injuries can and do occur in sports. Though you undoubtedly enjoy participating in athletics, you owe it to yourself to analyze the possible dangers involved in sports in order to best prepare yourself to prevent or deal with any problems.

Sports injury most often involves trauma. Trauma is injury due to mechanical and physical agents. In general medical classification, trauma injury falls into one of several descriptive categories: cuts, scrapes, contusions, ligament sprain, and muscular strain. Collectively, these conditions all possess one common distinction. Trauma in sports injury is the result of force.

Force is the functional result of mass and acceleration. Sudden stops and starts of projectiles (e.g. footballs, baseballs, etc.) or human body parts cause tremendous forces. And the magnitude of force is one determinant of the risk of possible injury.

The forces involved in human movement can be assessed with the aid of a force plate. This is a sensitive platform that is electronically connected to an oscilloscope. A force plate gives an accurate accounting of the forces involved as well as the time frame in which the forces occurred.

The other determinant of trauma is your body's ability to cope with those environmental forces with which it comes in contact. If environmental force exceeds the structural integrity of your body, something must tear or break.

From this discussion, it is now possible to suggest three general methods in which an athlete can minimize or prevent injury:

*This chapter is based upon material from the article, "Strength Training Called Baseball's Preventive Medicine," *Collegiate Baseball,* Vol. 24:6, March 20, 1981, pp. 9-10.

- Perfect the rules or techniques used in the game in order to reduce force.
- Use protective padding to absorb forces, thereby reducing them.
- Increase the structural integrity of the body to better enable it to accommodate force.

Sanctioned sports often take advantage of protective padding and safer playing rules whenever possible to prevent or minimize injury, but few coaches or players are aware that strength training is a viable though largely untapped preventive measure. This is true because so few participants realize the possible benefits of strength training.

If a muscle is trained in a high-intensity, low force, full-range manner, it grows and becomes stronger. Since the muscle is enveloped in a connective tissue sheath, this sheath must also grow with the muscle. The connective tissue in a muscle coalesces at both ends to form the tendon. And the tendon must therefore grow and strengthen. The tendon connects to bones about a joint, which is further connected to ligaments and capsular components. As a result, muscular strengthening MUST influence connective tissue integrity. The human body is the only "machine" that has the capability of repairing itself, and muscular growth is not an isolated event. It occurs synchronously with all other support tissues of your body. The human body does not allow disproportionate growth of support tissues.

Another point to consider in this regard is the condition that ligament, tendon, cartilagenous, and bony tissues mend and grow stronger very slowly. They respond very poorly to direct modalities intended to increase their protective margins. But muscle is a tissue that responds very quickly to exercise. Muscle will demonstrate a greater magnitude of growth in a shorter time than any other body tissue. Therefore, strength training is the surest and quickest method, though indirect, to effect support tissue enhancement. This is true when applied as a preventive or rehabilitative measure.

Since the introduction of high-intensity training techniques, preventive exercise has become a practical reality. This concept is indeed practical yet not practiced . . . Why?

Strength training PROVIDES the best prophylactic precaution available to the serious athlete. But proper strength-training principles are difficult to impose upon an athlete without taking human nature into account.

Sports medicine doctors and trainers often remark that many injuries might have been prevented or minimized if the athlete involved were only stronger. But the typical athlete becomes concerned and truly motivated toward strength training AFTER an injury. This is especially true on the professional level. Once an athlete is injured, possibly affecting the fate of his career and potential contract, he musters all that is within him to overcome defeat. But once a handsome contract is signed and in his hands, his interest in maintaining a high level of strength and personal fitness wanes again

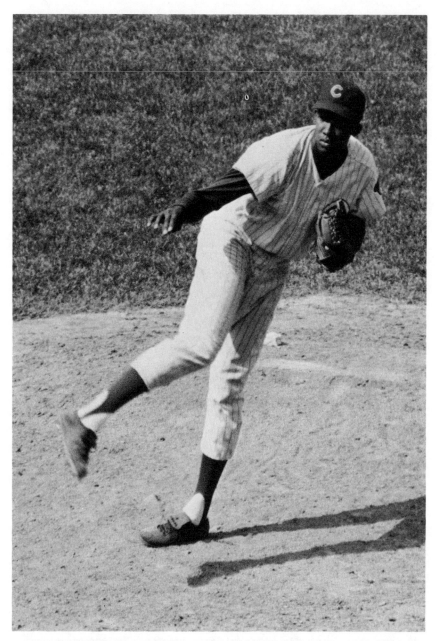

Many injuries might have been prevented or minimized if the athlete involved were only stronger. The typical athlete, however, becomes concerned and truly motivated toward strength training only after suffering an injury.

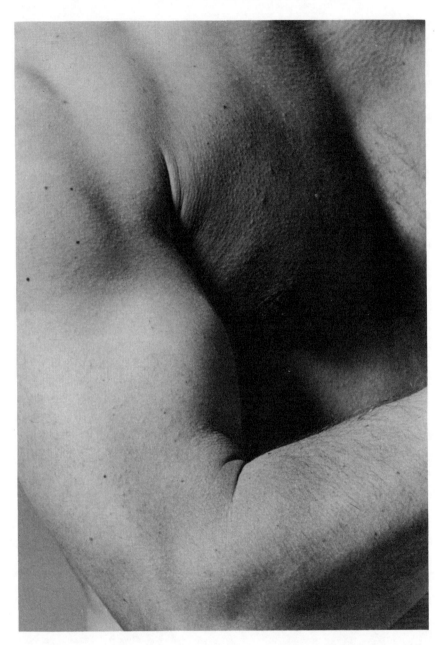

If a muscle is trained in a high-intensity, low-force, full-range manner, it grows and becomes stronger. The human body is the only "machine" that has the capability of repairing itself and muscular growth is not an isolated event. It occurs synchronously with all other support tissues of the body.

until the next catastrophe.

Such behavior is not unexpected. Proper strength training principles demand very hard and brief effort. For most people, serious training is not fun, comfortable, or pleasurable in any sense of the word. High-intensity exercise does not represent an easy road to success, but the benefits of strength training will make possible a better game, a safer game, and a more enjoyable game.

ABOUT THE EDITOR

James A. Peterson, PhD did his graduate work at The University of Illinois (Champaign) and his undergraduate work at The University of California (Berkeley). The author of seventeen books on sports and conditioning, Dr. Peterson was on the faculty of the United States Military Academy for nine years (1971-1980) where he served as the project director for a number of pioneer studies which investigated selected aspects of strength training methodology. During the 1981-82 academic year, he was employed as a consultant on fitness by The Stanford University Athletic Department. He and his wife Sue developed the entrance exam fitness test for The New York City Police Department and currently act as fitness consultants to a number of national organizations. At the present time, Dr. Peterson serves as the Director of Sports Medicine for the Women's Sports Foundation.